'In writing this book, [Rachel] has laid out a fund of knowledge on the brain and ADHD and translated it for parents and children affected. Reading this book will enable them to learn and put into practice the best available evidence. Rachel's book is…a book that everyone should read. … She explains the brain and the likely causes of its problems in easy language. But more than that, she provides nutritional advice for maintaining a healthy brain, which is what we all need… Rachel's book not only provides answers to what to do but even gives delightful recipes. She notes "Changing one's diet isn't easy, and Chapter 10 provides tools for making those changes, including a chart for meal planning." With mental ill-health on the rise, there is every good reason to read this book. It is with great pleasure that I recommend this book to all.'

– Professor Michael Crawford, PhD, FRSB, FRCPath

'I so admire Rachel. She has sacrificed a successful and lucrative career in real estate for the dubious delights of neuroscience research – insecure employment, ferocious competition, not to mention misogyny – in order to better understand and help ADHD. Using her formidable determination, intelligence and networking talents, she has overcome most of the obstacles thrown in her way to achieve the extraordinary understanding and practical helpfulness clinically that is shown in spades in this book.'

– Professor John Stein

'Rachel has been an invaluable guide for me as a mum to help me support my four very different boys. Her thinking outside of the box approach is way ahead of anything that is currently on offer for parents and once again highlights that what we feed our children has a direct impact on their behaviour and thinking and subsequently their lives. A must for any parent who is sick of the one-size-fits-all and outdated approach to nutrition we are still taught to accept.'

– Davinia Taylor, actor and biohacker and mum to four boys

'Good nutrition is a key tool in managing ADHD – this is the book we need!'

– Rory Bremner, British comedian

'This book teaches parents how to feed their family in very healthy and nutritious ways which may help support their learning and development as well as their mental health.'

– Dr Sara Taylor, clinical psychologist

'Rachel has been an absolute inspiration to me and helps me understand my ADHD through using different skills to embrace it and also to manage life on a day-to-day basis by eating specific foods and nutrients, especially omega-3 oils and less fatty and processed food. I am honoured to be the trust ambassador for Nutritious Minds, where I get to help people who suffer like me with mental health and by being part of such a phenomenal organization I get to not only pass a message and help others, I also help myself by doing this amazing work. I am so proud of the great work Dr Rachel Gow has done by letting people suffering know that it's not just about medication but also massively about the food we eat… I am proud to call her my friend.'

– Paul Danan, actor

'This book is simply a must-read for every parent. As a neuroscientist, clinical psychologist and parent, I am fully aware of how difficult it is to combine your expertise with your family life. The impact of nutrition on brain structure and function cannot be ignored, the consequences imply an enormous amount of stress and suffering for the individuals and their families. However, food industry interests seem to be too strong to fight against them. Rachel shows in her book how little nutritional value is in pre-processed food and drinks, how that is related to brain health, and provides us with easy and delicious recipes to enjoy family food in a healthy way. I can tell from experience my children love these recipes. Thanks Rachel!'

– Dr Ana Cubillo, clinical psychologist, neuroscientist and mother of two

Smart Foods for ADHD and Brain Health

of related interest

Can I Tell You About ADHD?
A Guide for Friends, Family and Professionals
Susan Yarney
Illustrated by Chris Martin
ISBN 978 1 84905 359 4
eISBN 978 0 85700 708 7

ADHD – Living without Brakes
Martin L. Kutscher
ISBN 978 1 84310 873 3
eISBN 978 1 84642 769 5

The Functional Nutrition Cookbook
Addressing Biochemical Imbalances Through Diet
Lorraine Nicolle and Christine Bailey
ISBN 978 1 78592 991 5
eISBN 978 0 85701 052 0

Food Refusal and Avoidant Eating in Children, including those with Autism Spectrum Conditions
A Practical Guide for Parents and Professionals
Gillian Harris and Elizabeth Shea
ISBN 978 1 78592 318 0
eISBN 978 1 78450 632 2

Smart Foods for ADHD and Brain Health

How Nutrition Influences Cognitive Function, Behaviour and Mood

Dr Rachel V. Gow

Forewords by Rory Bremner and Professor Robert H. Lustig

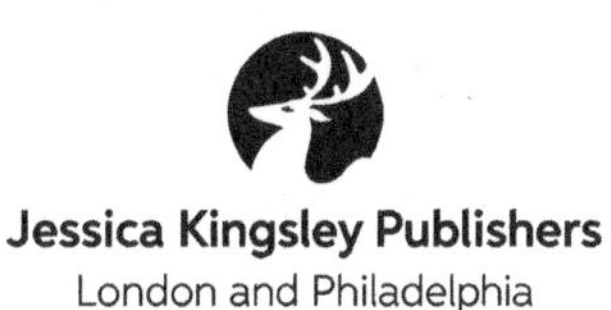

Jessica Kingsley Publishers
London and Philadelphia

First published in Great Britain in 2021 by Jessica Kingsley Publishers
An Hachette Company

7

A CIP catalogue record for this title is available from the British Library and the Library of Congress

ISBN 978 1 78592 446 0
eISBN 978 1 78450 821 0

Printed and bound by CPI Group (UK) Ltd, Croydon, CR0 4YY

Jessica Kingsley Publishers' policy is to use papers that are natural, renewable and recyclable products and made from wood grown in sustainable forests. The logging and manufacturing processes are expected to conform to the environmental regulations of the country of origin.

Jessica Kingsley Publishers
Carmelite House
50 Victoria Embankment
London EC4Y 0DZ

www.jkp.com

To my smart, creative and
most treasured children,
Esty and Nat.

To all parents of
neurodiverse children,
you are not alone.

Contents

RECIPES

Foreword

Rory Bremner, British comedian, diagnosed with adult ADHD

In life, as in comedy, timing is everything.

Rachel Gow's book comes at a time when mental health in general, and ADHD (Attention Deficit Hyperactivity Disorder) in particular, are at last receiving the kind of attention and understanding they deserve. In January 2018, the UK established the first All-Party Parliamentary Group on ADHD, to focus the attention of politicians and lawmakers on a condition that affects 1 in 20 of our children – 500,000 in the UK, or roughly one in every classroom. This is a breakthrough moment.

Children – and adults – with ADHD can be amongst the most creative, energetic, brilliant, positive and influential members of society. Yet, undiagnosed, misunderstood or stigmatized, they can all too easily 'fall through the cracks', their energy seen as disruptive, their frustration and despair driving them to the margins – self-diagnosing with drink or drugs, falling in with a bad crowd, moving from classroom to courtroom – and becoming one of the 30 per cent or so of the prison population that is estimated to be diagnosably ADHD.

This may all seem depressing, but the challenge is incredibly exciting. Just imagine the transformation we could make with better understanding, treatment and management of this condition – for society, of course, but most of all for the individuals concerned who are liberated, freed, able to realize their full potential.

And that potential is huge. Amongst the world's greatest athletes and artists you will find people whose ADHD made them who they are – restless, creative, determined, successful. Michael Phelps, Simone Biles, Justin Timberlake and will.i.am all acknowledge this.

I think of ADHD as my best friend and my worst enemy: worst enemy in the sense that it isn't always fun to be disorganized, forgetful, easily distracted, impulsive or manic with half-completed tasks and an impossible backlog of commitments; but best friend in that it makes me who I am. It allows me to make those leaps of imagination or random connections that fire my creativity and gives me the energy, and – an ADHD bonus – this gifts me the secret weapon of *hyperfocus*. This is when the ADHD brain is fully engaged on something which stimulates and rewards it, to the exclusion of everything else – distraction, discouragement, time itself.

What's it like inside that ADHD head? Imagine sitting in an open-plan office, your computer constantly showing alerts, your phone vibrating with notifications and texts, the person next to you (on either side) speaking on the phone, a television on the wall showing sports highlights or breaking news and a fire engine going past. That's what it's like inside an ADHD mind a lot of the time. So how extraordinary, then, that the engaged ADHD mind also has the ability to cast all that aside and hyperfocus intensely, if the task excites it. The potential is incredible.

And now, at last, we are beginning to move away from the stigmatic caricature of 'naughty children' and 'bad parents' towards an understanding that ADHD is a neurodevelopmental condition. Brain MRI (magnetic resonance imaging) scans show us that areas of the brain which regulate our impulsivity and help us prioritize, organize and function effectively and efficiently are significantly less developed in ADHD children. We know that in ADHD people, dopamine – that chemical, that neurotransmitter which stimulates and rewards the functioning brain – is not being released at typical levels.

To this improvement in knowledge and understanding we must add nutrition, which is where Rachel's book, and the research behind it, comes in. An understanding of the role nutrition plays in the development of our brains is so valuable. It gives us another weapon in the fight. It can positively influence the way our brains grow and develop.

And that, combined with other advances both in science and in understanding, is so exciting. I heartily welcome and recommend this book.

Foreword

Please Pay Attention

Professor Robert H. Lustig, MD, MSL

I don't have ADD (Attention Deficit Disorder), but I remember the first time I heard the term. It was a Friday morning in March 1982, I was a paediatric resident at St Louis Children's Hospital, and a visiting professor was giving Grand Rounds on this new disease state called 'Attention Deficit Disorder'. The idea of brain dysfunction leading to altered cognition and behaviour wasn't new. In fact, amphetamine in the 1930s and methylphenidate in the 1950s were used to treat what was then known as 'hyperkinetic impulse disorder' – emphasis on the 'hyperkinetic'. As I learned during my training, many of these early patients had other antecedents of brain dysfunction, such as perinatal asphyxia, cerebral palsy or brain tumours, or they were the offspring of alcohol or drug addicts. But then, in the early 1980s, kids were getting diagnosed with inattention, but without the hyperkinesis, and without any of the obvious antecedents. Is this a new disorder? What could be the cause? Why is this happening now? Why is the incidence increasing?

What was then an oddity is now fully 7.2 per cent of children and adolescents worldwide. However, there are hot spots of ADD. The UK has a 10 per cent prevalence, and the US is at 11 per cent, but with a wide range, from 5.6 per cent in Nevada to 18 per cent in Kentucky (Sayal *et al.* 2018). Moreover, ADD is not the only childhood mental health disorder. What about addiction, depression and anxiety? They've gone up on a parallel path in the paediatric age group, as their brains are still developing, and therefore are more vulnerable to all neurobehavioural disorders. Do you really think that a global insult affecting something as complex as the brain would only exhibit one symptom? And please let's not ignore the type 2 diabetes crisis that has overtaken the healthcare system of every civilized country, which started at the same time. So, what exposure started in developed countries in the late 1970s, and has migrated around the world, so that everyone in the world is now vulnerable?

You go up in your attic, and there's a wasp buzzing around. What are you going to do? Kill the wasp? Or get rid of the wasp nest? You have to work upstream of the problem if you are going to fix the cause. This is the challenge of public health. You know there's a root cause, but that cause may not be obvious. Treating the symptoms doesn't fix the cause. So what's the cause of our mental and metabolic health debacle? Can we identify what lies upstream and fix it before it is too late? Our survival as a society, and indeed as a species, depends on it.

The current UK and US prevalences of 10 per cent and 11 per cent for ADD and 8 per cent and 10.5 per cent for diabetes, mental and/or metabolic health disorders affect you directly (Diabetes UK 2020; Centers for Disease Control and Prevention 2020). Each of you either has ADD, has a child with ADD, or knows someone with ADD. And each of you has diabetes, has a parent with diabetes, or knows someone with diabetes. My daughter has ADD. Yes, knowing all that I know, she has ADD, I couldn't prevent it. And Rachel Gow's son has ADD. She gave up her previous life as a real estate agent because of it. Her son brought her to the science, and she's done it. She's got the degree, she's got the cred. She's my friend and colleague. And she is now one of the leading lights showing us the way out of this public health nightmare.

The short answer to the many questions raised – as globalization has spread, so has the consumption of palatable industrial foods. Food develops the brain. Food changes the brain. But unfortunately, food also poisons the brain. The study of this is part of the field of *nutritional psychiatry*. It also develops, changes and poisons the liver and pancreas. This is addressed by the field of *metabolic medicine*. Both used to be the province of quacks and touchy-feely granola types. But that was before the science. Now the science is in. You eat food, so does your kid, and what you eat is what your kid eats, so you are both study subjects. But that means you can fix yourself and your kid at the same time. I care. Rachel cares. You can't afford not to care. And that's why you must read this book, and then recommend it to anyone and everyone who still has a brain and a liver and a pancreas and who will listen.

Preface

My Story – From Real Estate Agent to Neuroscientist

Welcome to my book and wow, what a journey it has been so far! Thank you for picking it up, smart choice! I am so excited you selected to read this, not just because this book will help you heal your and your child's brain health, elevate your and their mood and teach you to adopt a mindful approach to all that you do – but because it is a sizeable reflection of the knowledge I have accumulated over the past 15 years during my journey from real estate agent to neuroscientist. Above all, the contents of this book permit careful reflection regarding where we are as a collective community in relation to brain health (this term replaces what is commonly referred to as mental health) versus where we need to be. It serves as a guide to make meaningful and positive changes in our own life, the lives of our loved ones and all those with neurodiverse conditions who struggle on a daily basis.

First, I would like to share with you how I came to end up working at one of the most respected medical research centres in the world: the National Institutes of Health (NIH) in Bethesda, Maryland, USA. Some of you may know that the NIH is an agency of the US Department of Health and Human Services that conduct high-risk, cutting-edge, novel research, and ultimately assists in the prevention and treatment of diseases. Its ground-breaking research and discoveries have contributed to saving and preventing suffering in countless human lives! It was an honour and a privilege to devote four years of my life to conducting the world's first neuroimaging trial testing the effects of omega-3 in the brain function of adults with Attention Deficit Hyperactivity Disorder (ADHD). This is an area of research I am immensely passionate about, and I will tell you why. My life monumentally changed direction in my mid-twenties because I was profoundly and personally affected by an experience that resulted in a choice to dedicate my life to advocating for brain health and neurodiverse conditions. My personal story and struggle forced me to adjust my sails and motivated me to commit to the course of helping others in the process.

Nathaniel

I was a young, working, first-time mother who adored my first-born son. He felt even more special because I had been adopted at the age of six months, and so I held onto him like the precious goods that he was. His name, Nathaniel, means *gift from God*, and I truly believed he was sent to me for a reason. However, very early on, my intuition told me that something might be *wrong* because although developmentally there were many similarities to other children of his age, the differences stood out. At three years of age, my little boy was bright, inquisitive and incredibly articulate. He had achieved all his milestones ahead of expectation, and as a pre-schooler, he could spell his nine-letter name aloud and even spoke a little French that I had taught him. Admittedly, he was cheeky, and a little naughty, but I preferred to think of his behaviour as simply mischievous. And yes, he could be hyperactive and a handful, but I attributed this as just a part of his playful personality.

Fast forward to the age of five and he would ask me things like, 'How does a light bulb work, Mummy?' He would spend time looking up the planets in the solar system and calling out their names – *Jupiter, Neptune, Pluto*. He learned which ones were closer to each other and then to Earth. I frequently didn't have the answers for his persistent scientific enquiries, and because of this I compensated by stacking his bookshelf full of adventures, fun facts and figures. Books pretty much fed his imagination and provided most of the answers to his questions. He loved everything, from Greek mythology to fairy tales by Hans Christian Andersen, Harry Potter to *Lord of the Rings* and, arguably his favourite, the *Guinness Book of Records*. At times, I felt ill equipped to cater for this beautiful, bright little boy with such boundless energy.

Looking back, there was no doubt that my son was noticeably restless, impulsive and hyperactive. He had struggled to sit still on the mat at nursery during story time for more than five minutes, and much to the great frustration of the teaching staff he would get up without permission and run around. When he started school his restless behaviour during lessons continued. The teachers categorized him with all sorts of labels – careless, disorganized, clumsy, naughty, lazy, a disruption – and told me that he didn't seem to learn from the consequences of his actions. All of this affected his self-esteem, and the more criticism he received, the more clowning around he did. Despite some noticeable underlying sadness, he remained very loving. I still remember him coming home after school with flower(s) he had picked (yes, unfortunately from other people's gardens!) and there was always an 'I love you, Mummy'.

The boys in his class knew exactly how to wind him up and then tell tales on him, so he would constantly get into trouble even if he hadn't actually committed the actual act he was accused of. The teasing could quickly escalate and become physical, which would inevitably result in him retaliating and pushing or punching them back, only to be caught and sent home for three days or longer. The adults told him, 'You should have told a teacher' and 'You need to think before you act'. However, this was all rather difficult advice to follow for an energetic, restless and impulsive little boy.

Marvel comic book heroes were one of my son's favourite 'obsessions', and Spider-Man was his childhood hero. It would not be unusual for my son to soar into the air or from sofa to table impersonating characters he admired without any fear of danger or the appropriateness or consequence of the situation. As you can imagine, it often ended in tears, and the saying *you need eyes in the back of your head* really did apply to me.

The accidents were frequent, from falling off swings and slides to 'Yabba dabba doooo-ing' through a glass coffee table during an episode of the Flintstones. And one day, he even swallowed a golden apple-shaped pendant from one of my necklaces! The X-ray was pretty hysterical, but what was not was having to monitor his bowel movements over the next 24 hours.

The Summons to See the Head Teacher

I think my life-changing moment came the day I was summoned to Nathaniel's primary school by his head teacher to *discuss his behaviour*. I can still recall the overwhelming and heart-sinking dismay I experienced when she told me, quite insensitively, that she thought he might be 'brain-damaged'. I left that meeting feeling utterly distraught; it was as if my entire world had collapsed. I suspect many other parents of neurodiverse children have experienced moments like these. Even if this is not the language I would have used myself, I think I did already know there was something different about Nathaniel. For a while I had not been quite ready to face up to the possibility that perhaps my son was different in some way.

At this time, I was a young, first-time mum, working long hours in the property field on Abbey Road, St John's Wood in North West London, near the famous EMI recording studios. I was juggling motherhood and work independently as a single mum, and the last straw was being asked to quietly remove my son from his private school in Abercorn Place, as the teachers couldn't cope with him. Desperate investigations into 'what was wrong' began, and over the years I sought guidance and answers, as so many of us have, from a wide range of professional services including educational psychologists, clinical psychologists, child psychiatrists, learning and behaviour coaches, mentors, nutritional specialists, and even chiropractors.

We tried everything, from allergy tests, to changing diets, methylphenidate, vitamin and omega-3 supplements as well as every after-school activity imaginable: athletics, martial arts, boxing, gymnastics, stage coach, trampolining, art and more.

My son was going to a new school where they had put great efforts into obtaining a statement of special educational needs (SEN) (now known as an Education Health Care Plan, EHCP, or an Individualized Education Plan, IEP, in the US) from the local education authority under the remit of 'emotional and behavioural difficulties' (EBD). To me, this was an unwanted label that explained nothing, but it would enable a small sum of money to be allocated to Nathaniel's local school so they could fund additional classroom support for him.

Eventually, after seeking several independent evaluations, we received diagnostic labels of 'mild Dyslexia' and probable ADHD. Receiving both diagnoses certainly helped me as a mother better validate and understand my son's behaviour. Yet, while I felt some relief and mild comfort, well-meaning friends and family members frequently challenged these diagnostic labels, telling me instead:

> 'It's not ADHD; he just needs more discipline.'
>
> 'If he were mine, I'd teach him not to misbehave.'
>
> 'ADHD? Isn't that just a funny made-up label for naughty kids?'

'That's not a real disorder though, is it?'

'He just needs a good smack.'

Sound familiar?!

Becoming an Expert

I found myself investigating these conditions better than an FBI agent! I had been thrown into a world that was entirely foreign and that came with a language I didn't fully understand. There were few signposts, and so, without the use of a compass, I had to learn to navigate through this new environment as best as I could, as many parents of children like Nathaniel do. We acquire a new style of speech – one of symptoms, assessments and diagnoses. We learn the processes of SEN statements and statutory assessments, the procedures of tribunals and educational law.

This was also an emotional journey, which I would describe as something like this: courage/despair; frustration/despair; hope/despair – each positive side by side with its opposing negative. As so many of us do, I felt a great need to become my own expert so I could, in turn, patiently explain the symptoms to unknowing teachers and other parents and professionals who were active and present in my son's life. Although ADHD is much more in the public eye now, there remain many misconceptions.

After much soul-searching I decided to give up my career in real estate and enrol in university. I was fortunate that I was granted entry under the criterion of 'mature student', and so I started a Bachelor of Science to study Psychology. Fast forward a monumental 10 years later, I emerged with three degrees, including a PhD, and sufficient expertise in ADHD, related behavioural differences and the knowledge that what you eat actually affects your brain function! Who would have thought?

A Book about ADHD, Brain Health and Diet

ADHD and other learning and behaviour differences are often called *neurodiverse* conditions, or referred to as *neurodiversity,* in reference to subtle differences in the wiring of the brain. Although some view these differences as a competitive advantage, ADHD in particular remains controversial. This is in spite of decades of genetic and neuroscientific evidence documenting the origin and course of its development, in addition to countless published journal articles of clinical trial data highlighting the importance of diet.

I believe that it is a great disservice that the condition remains misunderstood by the vast majority of people in a position to act positively – family practitioners, head teachers, school governors, social workers and other parents. Importantly, we need to recognize that these behavioural differences have their origin in the brain, not in bad parenting or some invisible devil perched on the child's shoulder, and the first step is understanding that the ability to improve our – and our children's – brain health is within our reach. It is a great honour to serve as your guide and to teach you how, through an evidence-based neuroscientific approach.

I learned initially by experimenting with foods at home, and then professionally during my academic career, that there are 'brain-selective' nutrients which are critical for the functioning of our brain, and which also help improve learning, mood and behaviour. When we eat smart and exercise, we feel great! Making nutritional changes is entirely within your reach as an individual, a parent or a professional advising parents. And it's a game-changer for overall health and happiness. Let's go get this!

Introduction

Parents and those who work with children or for the health of children have most likely had experiences of supporting children with Attention Deficit Hyperactivity Disorder (ADHD). One in twenty children are affected by this disorder. Yet, despite the prevailing tendency to medicate these children, my research has found, and in this book I argue, and I hope convince you, that managing ADHD doesn't necessarily have to mean prescriptions.

Prescription medications are often the first bandage placed over a wound, but in this book I show you how to seek – and find – natural and healthy solutions that don't solely involve ingesting more pharmaceuticals with their possible side effects. What few people – even medical professionals – know is that nutrition can be key in managing ADHD symptoms. I have witnessed, researched and recorded the effects of nutrition in children and adults with ADHD and similar conditions and it is time to share my knowledge with other parents and open-minded professionals.

A thoughtful diet can have an enormous impact on any child with ADHD, but there are few resources out there for parents and professionals who want to approach ADHD from a place other than prescriptions. *Smart Foods for ADHD and Brain Health* not only takes a nutrition-based look at ADHD and its management; it also offers a method for building a healthy diet that works for the children in your life.

For this method to work, there will need to be some education about the brain, so in Chapter 1 I will introduce you to brain basics and some of the documented differences between a 'normal' brain and the brain of someone with ADHD. Understanding these differences is key to understanding why nutrition can help manage ADHD symptoms. You can skip the technical bits, but if you are patient, you will learn some important science that will really inform your understanding of ADHD.

In Chapter 2 I talk about the connection between the brain and the stomach, and how the health of one affects the other. The environment of the gut can have effects on learning, memory, mood and stress responses – all factors in ADHD symptoms. Gastrointestinal issues are more common in people who experience brain disorders, which shows that the gut–brain axis is something worth paying attention to. Learning how food can affect the brain will help you make conscious and more deliberate choices about how you feed a child's brain.

As Chapter 3 addresses, treating the ADHD brain isn't just about providing the right foods; it's also about avoiding the wrong ones. While pharmaceuticals have their place, food is also a powerful medicine. For example, early nutritional intervention in pregnancy with an emphasis on omega-3 fatty acids to optimize the health of the developing brain and potentially safeguard against some neurodevelopmental conditions such as ADHD. Food has been used for healing and medicinal purposes throughout history, but as we have further developed food with artificial flavouring, colouring, preservatives and additives, it can sometimes be a poison. In this chapter I show how, much like medications – including those for ADHD – certain foods can also have negative side effects, and exacerbate ADHD symptoms.

Nutrition is perhaps one of the easiest factors to control, but genetics also plays a role in ADHD. In Chapter 4 I talk about genetics and how even genes have some room for manipulation. Nutrition is one biological mechanism that may have the ability to turn certain aspects of genes on and off. This means that not only do food choices impact children on the gut–brain axis, but also at a cellular level, even post-birth.

Omega-3 fatty acids are amongst the most critical nutrients during foetus development and beyond birth for a healthy brain. However, omega-3 fatty acids are in direct competition with omega-6 fatty acids for receptors in the brain. The omega-6 to omega-3 ratio in a typical diet is not ideal, so it's important to not only increase omega-3 fatty acids, but also to decrease omega-6 intake. In Chapter 5, I will explain the conversion of short-chain polyunsaturated fatty acids (SC-PUFAs) into long-chain highly unsaturated fatty acids (LC-HUFAs). This knowledge is especially crucial for those who choose a vegan diet, as fish is the easiest source of omega-3.

Although omega-3 fatty acids are the big fish in combating ADHD with nutrition, there are other nutrient deficiencies that can increase the symptoms of ADHD. Knowing a child's vitamin and mineral levels allows for conscientious supplementation, especially for iron, zinc, magnesium, and vitamins D, B2, B6 and B9. Chapter 6 will describe the roles these nutrients play in children and in ADHD, along with ways for supplementing any that might be lacking.

Guiding a child into healthy eating means also taking into account food allergies and sensitivities. Chapter 7 addresses the difference between an intolerance and an allergy, as well as ways to spot the symptoms of each. Studies show that food intolerances can lead to attention issues, tantrums, irritability and other neurodiverse symptoms. Therefore, understanding a child's sensitivities will help build a diet for success.

The same foods and additives that may cause problems for children with ADHD have been shown to produce ADHD symptoms in children even without the disorder. Knowing what those foods are is critical, and understanding how food works in the body and brain can be extremely helpful. Chapter 8 goes more in-depth into the sugars and dyes in food that may cause attention problems in all children.

There are many diets already out there – ketogenic, Mediterranean, Feingold, etc. – but not all of these diets are helpful in managing ADHD symptoms. Chapter 9 looks at some of these diets, and other dietary habits that can help or hinder those with ADHD. There is also more information on the vegan diet and how to work within that for ADHD.

Mindfulness is seeing a lot of attention these days, but bringing it into a child's diet is something that might not occur to those managing ADHD. Changing one's diet isn't easy, and Chapter 10 provides tools for making those changes, including a chart for meal planning.

Following this chapter is a final section of delicious and healthy recipes and snacks that will help you construct a diet for not only managing ADHD symptoms but improving brain function and mental wellness.

You don't have to read the whole book before you can get started. At the end of each chapter is a 'Chapter Takeaway' that will hit the highlights of the chapter for you, as well as a 'Take a Step' section that gives a suggestion for implementing the knowledge of the chapter right away in one small way. The recipes can be a great way to take those steps.

The research and information in *Smart Foods for ADHD and Brain Health* provide a deeper understanding of the ADHD brain. Included in each chapter are messages from ADHD professionals, people with ADHD and/or parents. This book will give you the tools to develop a diet for any child with ADHD and the understanding to approach an alternative solution with confidence.

Chapter 1

The Brain and the ADHD Brain

In this chapter, I introduce you to brain basics and the main functional differences between a 'normal' brain and the brain of someone with ADHD. Understanding these differences is key to understanding why nutrition works as a treatment for ADHD symptoms. You can skim over or skip entirely the technical bits, but if you are patient, you will learn some important science that will really inform your understanding of ADHD, and you will get more out of the later chapters in the book.

The brain is home to who we are: our personalities and our minds. It defines us and governs our ability to make decisions, generate new ideas, act on or withhold our impulses, and experience deep emotional pleasure or pain.

Distinct from other organs, the frontal lobes of the brain take at least until early adulthood to fully mature, which explains a lot, especially in children with neurodevelopmental differences such as ADHD. This magnificent organ has enabled the human race to become the dominant species on Earth and is responsible for all our ground-breaking advances in technology, science and medical discoveries. The brain is the facilitator of language, which has given us the ability to evolve, communicate, exchange ideas and artefacts, and critically, to be sociable.

There should be no doubt that the human brain is one of the most critical and intricate organs in the body, a sophisticated maze of pathways, networks and regions, and yet, basic concepts about its structure and function are not well understood. As children we are taught about the workings of the human body – about the respiratory system and that our lungs help us breathe; that our heart pumps blood around the body, which keeps us alive; that bones and muscles enable us to function physically – but I would hedge a bet that an 11-year-old leaving primary school wouldn't be able to tell me about the function of the cerebellum.

When visiting children in schools, and teaching undergraduate and postgraduate students, I like to ask people what they think their brain is made up of – not a trick question, but genuinely because the majority of people on reflection are a little unsure. The answer 'fat' often comes as a great surprise.

I'll be talking a lot about healthy omega-3 fats in the following pages and the critical role that one of those fats – docosahexaenoic acid (DHA) – plays in both the structure and function of our brain and vision. Fats historically have been given a bad name, and the negative connotations of fats still exist to this day, quite simply because some so-called experts got it wrong, which resulted in dietary recommendations to eat low-fat foods. This book will set you straight, and by the end you will understand the different types of fats – that they are not a single entity that can be grouped together – and that omega-3 fats are absolutely brain-essential! Before we get into all of that, it will be helpful to understand what it is exactly that we are trying to nourish and nurture, so first let's learn a little more about the brain.

Brain Anatomy

There are many resources out there for a more thorough understanding of the brain's anatomy, but we are going to keep things simple here.

The brain contains a left and a right hemisphere that are separated by a thick bundle of nerve fibres. These send messages and permit communication between the left and right parts of the brain. This nerve bundle is not fully developed until puberty – hence the vital role played by 'brain foods' in a child's diet – and there are differences in size which are linked with sex, handedness and conditions such as schizophrenia and Dyslexia. However, not all the studies in this area are consistent, and so the significance of this is debatable (Beaumont, Kenealy and Rogers 1991).

The oldest, most primitive part of the brain is called the brainstem. This contains the medulla (which means 'long marrow' in Latin) and is critical for controlling respiration and cardiac function. The next region is the pons (Latin for 'bridge'), spinal cord and cerebellum ('little brain'). The cerebellum is involved in movement, posture and the automatic elements of, for example, throwing a ball. It is also linked to attention processes and some types of learning (Wickens 2004).

The forebrain (also known as the diencephalon) is the largest part of the brain, positioned anteriorly, and plays a key role in the processing of complex cognitive functions. It has a bulbous part which surrounds the older 'tubular brain'. The forebrain contains both cerebral hemispheres, the thalamus (Greek for 'inner chamber') and the hypothalamus (meaning 'under the thalamus'). The thalamus has regions that transmit information related to sight and sound. The hypothalamus is part of the limbic system; it is an extremely old structure, and one we share with many members of the animal kingdom. In humans it is only about the size of a grape, and yet it is linked to a wide range of behaviours including feeding, sex, biological rhythms, reinforcement, emotion and aggression. The hypothalamus is continuously supervising the internal workings of our bodies, and with this information, making necessary motivational or behavioural adjustments. The hypothalamus also controls the regulation of the 'autonomic nervous system' and the release of hormones, including dopamine, from the pituitary gland (Wickens 2004).

The remainder of the forebrain is called the endbrain (or telencephalon), and it contains the cerebral cortex. This is considered the part of the brain that makes us uniquely human – it is the site of the mind (or consciousness, if you like) and is involved in aspects of memory, learning, language, movement, touch and vision. It also plays an important role in helping us plan and organize, think ahead, understand the consequences of our actions and engage in abstract thought. In other words, exactly what you are doing now reading this – thinking about and understanding the function of the brain. It is also quite deceptive, as it appears much smaller than it actually is. In fact, if you were to unfold and flatten it out, its surface area would map out to be approximately 75cm^2.

Next is the cerebral cortex, which contains four lobes: frontal, parietal, temporal and occipital, each of which I briefly explain.

The frontal lobes are the last parts of the brain to mature and are normally fully developed around mid-adulthood, between the ages of 23 and 25. This is in contrast to the oldest, reptilian part of our brain, called the limbic system, which generates primal emotions such as anger and rage, and in this context can be thought of metaphorically as the accelerator. The frontal lobes are involved in judgement, decision-making, problem-solving, memory, language, spontaneity, initiation, impulse control, and social and sexual behaviour. They are responsible for what is described as executive function (EF), including self-regulation, that is, motor and interference inhibition control, attention control (selective and sustained attention), forethought, planning, delay of gratification, working memory, problem-solving and cognitive flexibility

(Baddeley 1996; Stuss and Alexander 2000). It is helpful to think of the frontal lobes of the brain as the cognitive brakes, reining in irrational or illogical impulses, urges and desires. An impaired frontal cortex may result in less cognitive control over the limbic system, leading to a reduction in self-control, a greater addiction to risk and poor problem-solving skills (Casey, Jones and Hare 2008).

The parietal lobes are linked to attention – in particular, the ability to pay attention for prolonged periods of time – novel or distracting stimuli, including sudden changes in sensory stimulation, and the process of becoming familiar with an object or situation. Some areas of the parietal lobes are also linked to language.

The temporal lobes are primarily involved in hearing and the processing of sound in order to transform it into meaningful things such as speech and words, enabling us to understand spoken language. The temporal lobes also play a key role in the formation of long-term memory.

The occipital lobes are concerned with processing and encoding information from the visual system and transmitting it to adjacent cortical regions. These include separate cortical areas involved in spatial awareness, reading, object recognition, colour and movement.

The brain's regions work in synergy with each other. They are not isolated structures, and like a computer, they are also vulnerable to malfunction. In fact, neuroscientific research has taught us that the brain is susceptible to a wide range of environmental factors, including nutrition, exercise and sleep deprivation, hormonal imbalances and poor physical health, as well as toxicity and infection.

ADHD

In the clinical literature, neurodiversities originate as a result of subtle differences occurring during development in the wiring and structure of the brain that can give rise to alterations in cognitive and emotional functions. As the foetal brain is developing, it is sensitive to many internal and external factors that may hamper development. These include genetic and metabolic diseases, immune disorders, infectious diseases, deprivation, physical trauma, toxicity, environmental factors and nutritional insufficiencies. Any interruption in neurodevelopment as a result of these factors may result in slight deviations in the wiring of the brain, increasing risk for a neurodevelopmental condition, the most common of which is ADHD. ADHD overlaps and has shared features with other neurodevelopmental conditions, such as Autism Spectrum Disorder (ASD), Foetal Alcohol Spectrum Disorder (FASD), Developmental Coordination Disorder (DCD) and communication, speech and language disorder (Dyslexia).

The classic textbook explanation defines ADHD as one of the most pervasive psychiatric disorders of childhood. However, I am less concerned with diagnostic labels than with the actual features – the learning and behavioural differences.

There are three recognized subtypes of ADHD:

- Predominantly inattentive (Attention Deficit Disorder, ADD) (includes disorganization).
- Predominantly hyperactive-impulsive.
- Combined presentation: inattentive and hyperactive-impulsive (ADHD).

It is estimated that ADHD affects between 6 and 13 per cent of the worldwide population. It has been suggested that it exists primarily in the West (e.g. the US, the UK, European Union (EU) member states, Canada, Australia, New Zealand and parts of Latin America). This is not actually the case, although it is perhaps more likely to be recognized and diagnosed in Western medicine. Scientific studies have reported ADHD as existing cross-culturally in nations including Africa, Asia, Thailand, Jamaica, South America, the Middle

East and Japan, to name just a few (Moffitt and Melchior 2007). The condition is reported to affect more males than females, at a ratio of 4:1, but this is hypothesized to be because boys manifest more overt features of ADHD, such as higher levels of hyperactive and impulsive behaviours, while girls are more likely to have the head-in-the-clouds, daydreamer, inattentive traits associated with the ADD subtype.

Olivia Grant, Actor with ADHD, Daughter of Carrie Grant

Friedrich Wilhelm Nietzsche once said, 'those who were seen dancing were thought to be insane by those who could not hear the music'.

Having ADHD in this society crushes your self-confidence. I spent my school life judging my shortcomings against neurotypical people. I wasn't the hyper kid, or the naughty kid, so when I first heard the term 'ADHD' being used to reference me, I was confused because that was all I had ever learned that ADHD was.

Getting my diagnosis five years ago when I was 18 was the most freeing and liberating thing. I finally understood why I am the way I am, and that the way I am is brilliant. I am scatty, my brain races, I'm anxious a lot of the time, I used to be really disorganized, I'm now hyper organized – it lowers my anxiety. It sometimes takes me a bit longer to do the process of hearing someone, understanding what they've said and then replying. I have a deficit in my attention span, unless I am hooked in to what I'm doing – and then I am more focused than you could ever imagine. My art and creativity is the way I have learned to channel the inner impulsivity and brain racing; I'm always writing, singing, acting and constantly finding new ways to express my creativity through art.

When I look at some of my friends who to me are clearly ADHD but don't have a diagnosis, it's so hard to watch, because they could be so much freer than they are. Instead, they beat themselves up for not being able to achieve certain things, they self-medicate, and the hardest thing is that they don't have an understanding of what ADHD actually is because the actual traits have never been explained to them. We have a long way to go to catch up.

I fear for the parents who live with daily judgement, who feel they are continually failing to live up to the impossible standard of producing cookie-cutter children. I fear for the lost generation of men and women sitting in prisons or with mental health issues or just not following their dreams because no one ever noticed their brains were just wired differently, no one ever took the time to nurture those people's specific wondrous strengths. If they had been given understanding, if they had been encouraged in school, I truly believe it could have made all the difference. I fear for the next generation going through school right now. We need to make sure it will be different for them.

I wish that going through school someone had told me that it was okay to have a brain that is wired differently, that my strengths, although they look different, are just as valuable. I have learned the brilliance in brains that work differently, that diversity of thinking is what shapes society. We need the ones who see the world differently to make the world different, to make the world the best it can be.

Common behavioural problems attached to ADHD can drive parents and teachers wild. I know as I have experienced them first-hand, both at home in my family life and during my work with families with ADHD. They may vary in form and nature but can include attention-seeking behaviour such as adopting the role of the classroom clown, unprovoked explosive meltdowns (especially in public spaces such as shopping malls, which is always a fun one!), repetitive behaviours, excessive talking and low-level disruptive behaviours such as tapping, not remaining seated, fidgeting and general restlessness. Symptoms of ADHD can even include the concept of hyperfocusing: an ability to shut out the outside world and focus intensely on a task or activity of great interest.

Children with ADD (the predominantly inattentive subtype of ADHD) struggle in a different way. These children are perpetually distracted – any noise or occurrence going on around them can cause significant distraction, drawing their attention away from their schoolwork. They then struggle to refocus back to the task at hand. The distraction can be something as simple as a loose cotton thread on their clothing, dry skin on their hand that simply has to be picked at, or other irrelevant stimuli. They can lose all concept of time and will struggle to organize themselves, instead losing items frequently and failing to finish tasks both at home and school without close supervision. Often these children appear not to be listening even when spoken to directly, causing frustration in both parents and teachers.

ADHD has previously been described by those who have it as an invisible condition because of the way it impacts brain function, which then manifests in problematic action and impulsive behaviour. What is meant by invisible is that other people don't instantly or easily recognize the symptoms. The problem with these 'invisible' symptoms is that, unlike Autism, the symptoms are not immediately obvious and are therefore less tangible and so vulnerable to criticism and false conclusions. When people challenge me on whether ADHD is even a real condition, naturally I share with them all the neuroscientific and genetic evidence I have acquired during my professional training, but I also challenge them to work or live with a child with ADHD for one month and then reengage in the conversation with me.

Contrary to popular belief, ADHD is not a new phenomenon nor is it a label simply made up in the 21st century. Although the concept of ADHD as defined by the *Diagnostic and Statistical Manual for Mental Illness* is relatively new, excessively hyperactive, inattentive and impulsive children have been described in medical literature since the late 18th century.

Sir Alexander Crichton, a Scottish physician, studied many cases of insanity and mental illness, and in 1798 described the first example of attention deficit in his second book, *On Attention and Its Diseases*. Crichton describes this as 'the incapacity of attending with a necessary degree of constancy to any one object'.

About a hundred years later, the German physician Heinrich Hoffmann (1809–1894) documented a case report of a young boy showing symptoms of hyperactivity, impulsivity and inattention. As well as being a physician, Hoffman was a gifted illustrator, and he captured the spirit of ADHD in a series of animated drawings about a boy he named 'Fidgety Philip' in his book *Der Struwwelpeter*:

> But fidgety Philip,
> He won't sit still;
> He wriggles,
> And giggles,
> And then, I declare,
> Swings backwards and forwards,
> And tilts up his chair,
> Just like any rocking-horse –
> 'Philip! I am getting cross!'
> See the naughty, restless child
> Growing still more rude and wild,
> Till his chair falls over quite.

Philip screams with all his might,
Catches at the cloth, but then
That makes matters worse again.
Down upon the ground they fall,
Glasses, plates, knives, forks, and all.
How Mamma did fret and frown,
When she saw them tumbling down!
And Papa made such a face!
Philip is in sad disgrace.

In 1851, Hoffmann rejected the notion that patients had criminal or obsessive tendencies, and viewed them simply as having psychiatric disorders in the same way as medical patients. Over two centuries later, most parents of children with ADHD can recognize traits in Fidgety Philip as the hyperactive-impulsive subtype of ADHD. Numerous other papers, studies and lectures through the centuries have noted hyperactivity in children and possible educational difficulties because of differences in the brain, including Franz Kramer's 'Hyperkinetic conditions in children', 'Symptoms and course of a hyperkinetic disease in children' and 'Psychopathic constitutions and organic brain diseases as causes for educational difficulties', throughout the 1930s (see Lange *et al.* 2010).

The ADHD Brain

This early research also uncovered potential links between physical brain differences and hyperactivity symptoms. Physical, observable brain characteristics were suspected to be related to hyperactivity. If you think of the analogy of the brain as a type of supercomputer with hardware (the brain structure) and software (the function leading to our behaviour), then any hardware problems can impact the software – causing it to fail to function exactly the way it should.

Research in the 1930s and 1940s had supported a link between brain injury and deviant behaviour. It was not just children with brain injuries who had developed behaviour disorders, but also those who had been exposed to infections and lead toxicity, as well as those with epilepsy (Lange *et al.* 2010). Around the same time, researchers were aware that monkeys who had been exposed to the surgical removal of their frontal lobe tissue displayed similar behaviour disturbances to hyperactive children (Barkley 2014). As stated earlier, the frontal lobes help govern our everyday behaviour, thoughts and actions. This experiment with monkeys suggested that frontal lobe damage might be linked to child hyperactivity.[1]

The notion of the brain-injured child first came into focus in the 1940s, and this eventually evolved into the concept of 'minimal brain damage' (Barkley 2014). For a long time, the consensus was that even if minimal damage to the brain could not be observed objectively, it could be witnessed behaviourally via overt hyperactivity, and could therefore be assumed to be present (Lange *et al.* 2010). Dr Maurice Laufer, of the International Institute on Child Psychiatry in Toronto, Canada, felt the term was limiting (Laufer, Denhoff and Solomons 1957). Dr Laufer was convinced that some children who met the criteria for the *hyperkinetic impulse* disorder did not have any record of traumatic or infectious factors in their histories. He used electrophysiological recordings (*electroencephalography,* EEG) to argue this point by measuring brain activity after a dose of the stimulant drug metrazol between children with and without hyperkinetic disorder. He found that after taking the drug the children with the *hyperkinetic impulse* subtype had responses that were now similar to that of the healthy control children (Lange *et al.* 2010).

This led Dr Laufer and his colleagues to consider that rather than brain damage, the children had functional disturbances of the

---

1 Experimental research commonly follows from the early cell culture laboratory studies to animals and then to humans. These are phases from bench to bedside, if you like. Ethics would not permit this type of research in humans, and all of the omega-3 deprivation studies are in animals or cell cultures.

forebrain (which includes the thalamus, hypothalamus, posterior portion of the pituitary gland, and pineal gland, an area key to releasing dopamine), and that this was the origin of hyperkinetic impulse disorder (Lange *et al.* 2010).

We have learned so much more about the brain during the past three decades, and much of that has been due to technological advances in neuroimaging techniques, which have permitted incredible new insights into the brain's structure and function, allowing clinical comparisons in ways that were previously not possible. Facilitated by the advancement of neuroscience, impairments in specific brain networks involving the prefrontal and striatal regions were proposed in children with ADHD compared to children without ADHD (Cubillo *et al.* 2011b). Furthermore, this imaging research linked abnormalities in the structure, volume (size) and function of the brain to ADHD and many other mental disorders (Hoogman *et al.* 2017; Shaw 2013).

A great deal of the functional neuroimaging research in the UK in ADHD has been led by Professor Katya Rubia and her colleagues at King's College London. Rubia's team have published several findings demonstrating consistent impairments within certain parts of the brain (the fronto-striatal and fronto-parietal circuits) in relation to inhibitory control (i.e. the ability to suppress or withhold a response), working memory (e.g. the ability to hold digits in the memory for short periods of time), and selective and sustained attention (Rubia 2007, 2018; Rubia *et al.* 2005).

The discovery and implementation of MRI (magnetic resonance imaging) has allowed scientists to view slices of the brain and surrounding tissue via the use of a strong magnet, a radio frequency (RF) transmitter, a receiver (antenna) and a computer for processing the received signal (Woolsey, Hanaway and Gado 2013). Functional magnetic resonance imaging (fMRI) is well suited for exploring neurofunctional processes that underlie the performance and behavioural differences in conditions such as ADHD and

Autism. Through neuroimaging we can establish which regions of the brain are activated during a resting state, or during tasks that measure processes related to memory, motivation, reward, inhibition (i.e. suppressing responses), emotions and so much more. Differences in some of these tasks have been found in individuals with ADHD compared to undiagnosed controls (Cubillo *et al.* 2009, 2011a; Rubia 2011).

The default mode network (DMN) of the brain measures the passive activity of the brain when it is at rest but is recalling past memories, emotions and autobiographical information, and when it is projecting into the future and piecing together stories – in other words, what the brain is doing when the person is not engaged in any particular task. This network can be viewed and its activity measured with an fMRI. The DMN shows increased or decreased levels of activity during this period, and is frequently more active in patients with depression and ADHD during rest and decreased during task-directed activities (Cortese *et al.* 2012). This decrease in DMN activity potentially illustrates why people with ADHD struggle to focus on task-directed activities. In a similar fashion, this pattern of DMN activity may also help to explain why people with ADHD and depression ruminate and struggle to switch off and/or calm intrusive thoughts when they are at rest. Professor Philip Asherson and his research team have linked the concept of spontaneous mind wandering to ADHD (Bozhilova *et al.* 2018) and this concept is hypothesized to reflect dysfunctional connectivity between executive control networks and the brain's DMN (Fox *et al.* 2015; Sripada 2014).

Tasks measuring EF have been investigated in children and adolescents with ADHD, and performance has shown significant differences compared to age-matched controls (Overtoom *et al.* 2002; Willcutt *et al.* 2005). In addition, low omega-3 has been related to differences in emotion processing and higher levels of callous and unemotional traits (Gow *et al.* 2013a, b). However, EF deficits alone are neither sufficient nor necessary for the presence of ADHD.

Brain Fat

It is pretty remarkable that a mass of fatty jelly is able to govern our everyday thoughts, behaviours and actions. If you held an adult human brain in your hands it would actually be quite heavy, weighing approximately 1.4kg, and oily to touch. The brain is, in fact, the fattiest organ in the human body. At least 65 per cent of its dry weight is made from specialized and complex fats called lipids, and around 25 per cent of all neuronal membranes are made of omega-3 fats. One of the singularly most important omega-3 fats present in the brain is docosahexaenoic acid, or DHA, which can be obtained by eating fish and seafood.

DHA is vital to communication throughout the brain. Each of the neurons in our brain contains an axon that passes messages away from the cell body to other neurons. These send an electric signal or impulse which then travels down the axon. Each axon is covered in a fatty sheath called myelin, which is made up of DHA. This brain-essential fat helps speed up cell signalling, resulting in speedy communication across our brain networks. Without adequate daily intakes of DHA the chemical messaging process would be less efficient and slower.

Nutritional insufficiencies during pregnancy can negatively impact both brain structure and function, which research findings have shown can predispose children to risk factors for antisocial behaviour (Adrian 2008; Liu 2011) and antisocial personality disorder in adulthood (Neugebauer, Hoek and Susser 1999), as well as posing a significant risk factor for increased aggressive and conduct-disordered behaviour in childhood and adolescence (Liu *et al.* 2004). Babies born prematurely have a higher requirement for DHA as they are denied the rapid accumulation that occurs during the third trimester (Makrides and Uauy 2014). Scientists have now suggested that the increased risks associated with preterm babies, such as global developmental delay and ADHD (Gow and Hibbeln 2014), may be partly linked to a fatty acid deficiency in utero. Furthermore, babies born prematurely have an increased risk of problems with vision, including premature retinopathy (a disease which leads to impaired vision) (Hellström, Smith and Dammann 2013) and Dyslexia (Stein 2001). If this one lack plays a role in neurodevelopmental conditions, it's no wonder that they sometimes overlap.

Professor John Stein, Neuroscientist, University of Oxford

I'm extremely honoured to have been asked to contribute to Rachel's book on ADHD. I've always admired her courage and determination in abandoning a secure and lucrative career in real estate in favour of a totally insecure and poorly paid vocation in research psychology and neuroscience, in pursuit of trying to help people with ADHD.

I first met Rachel through Eric Taylor, Emeritus Professor of Child and Adolescent Psychiatry at King's College London and Michael Crawford, Visiting Professor in the Department of Metabolism, Digestion and Reproduction at Imperial College London, who told me about her plans for an extremely ambitious PhD. I must confess that I was rather sceptical at first. She had actually already recruited a reasonably large number, nearly 100, of participants with ADHD, and she hoped to correlate their blood levels of omega-3 fatty acids not only with their ADHD symptoms, but also with their memory performance and emotional reactions, together with any differences in EEG responses from controls, and to cap it all, she wanted to carry out a randomized controlled trial of supplementing their diets with omega-3s to see if the adverse correlations could be reversed. Any one of these, particularly the last, would be a very large undertaking. But to achieve all of them in a mere three years with hardly any background in biochemistry, electrophysiology or the mysterious world of randomized controlled trials… Well…! In the event, however, my scepticism was totally misplaced. She pulled off most of her aims in a remarkable PhD, which I had the honour to examine and found very interesting.

My other reason for always watching Rachel's work is that my research with dyslexic children had convinced me that there is a huge overlap between Dyslexia (my first engagement with neurodevelopmental disorders) and ADHD. Indeed, recent surveys have shown the overlap to be over 50 per cent, and it's almost entirely an accident of which professional you first see as to whether you get diagnosed as Dyslexic or ADHD. Hence in our clinics for Dyslexia we see many children who could equally be diagnosed as ADHD. In all of them their most prominent symptoms are their problems with attention and being able to concentrate on anything for any length of time.

Having discovered in the 1970s that the cerebellum receives an important projection from the visual cortex of signals about the timing of visual events in the outside world that are provided by the visual 'magnocellular' system, I later developed the 'magnocellular theory' of Dyslexia. This postulates that defective neural timing, mediated by magnocells, underlies dyslexics' problems with sequencing letters and sounds properly. We also discovered that these magnocells' timing functions are highly dependent on an adequate supply of the omega-3 long-chain polyunsaturated fatty acid (LC-PUFA), docosahexaenoic acid (DHA), which enables their rapid responses. We found that giving our dyslexics DHA supplements usually improved their m-cell function and helped them to improve their reading. But the most striking effect of the omega-3 supplements was that their main effect seemed to be to help the children improve their attention and concentration.

Since one thing that I haven't managed to achieve yet is to convince Rachel of the mechanism whereby both Dyslexia and ADHD symptoms may be improved by omega-3s, my small contribution to her book is this belated attempt to do so.

How do omega-3s work? People tend to be very vague when trying to answer this question – they suggest that somehow omega-3s improve neuronal membrane structure, or that they're anti-inflammatory, or that they may have some exotic role in synaptic transmission. What we should concentrate on here, however, is to consider what is common to both ADHD and Dyslexia that might be helped by omega-3 supplements. In fact, the main problem with Attention Deficit Disorder (ADD), whether with or without hyperactivity, is, of course, an inability to control attention properly, so probably this is what we improve in children with either ADHD or Dyslexia or both, when we give them omega-3 supplements.

Recently, by combining results from fMRI, DTI (diffusion tension imaging), MEG (magnetoencephalography), EEG and graph theory computer modelling, much more has been learned about the brain differences that are responsible for the inattention in ADHD. In summary, the ADHD brain has been shown to be characterized by superior local connectivity, but inferior long-range connectivity, particularly in the dorsolateral prefrontal cortex, the area that usually takes control of one's voluntary allocation of attention and the ability to concentrate. This local hyper-connectivity coupled with distant hypo-connectivity in ADHD is indirectly demonstrated by an increased ratio of theta (θ) to beta (β) power (TBR) in their EEG recordings. Probably the locally well-connected modules tend to 'free wheel' and fail to communicate properly with their distant cousins to the detriment of their β phase locking; this may compromise the children's ability to concentrate.

Rachel showed that this β reduction is associated with lower plasma DHA in ADHD boys, while others have shown that this lack of DHA is particularly prominent in the prefrontal cortex. Thus incorporation of DHA into the brain, particularly the prefrontal cortex, appears to be much reduced in ADHD.

The crucial importance of DHA for the rapid timing of events in the brain has been demonstrated most directly by correlating the amount of DHA in the umbilical cord of newly born babies with the latency of their cortical EEG responses to a moving stimulus: the lower their cord DHA was, the more slowly their visual magnocellular signals about the motion reached the visual cortex. In ADHD children with low DHA, therefore, responses are slower, probably throughout the whole brain, reaching their nadir in the prefrontal cortex.

Gathering all these threads together, we can speculate that the reason why DHA supplements can help both dyslexic and ADHD children is that their incorporation into the membranes and synapses of magnocellular timing neurons speeds up their responses, and that this improves their long-range communications between local modules in the brain. This combats their tendency to phase-lock poorly, and thus facilitates the rapid but precisely timed shifts of attention that are required for optimum executive control of attention, and are so clearly lacking in those with ADHD.

I hope this convinces you, Rachel!

A body of research has demonstrated that the development and growth of connections between brain pathways is hindered in animals deprived of DHA, children and adolescents born preterm, and patients with psychiatric disorders including ADHD and bipolar disorder (McNamara 2006; McNamara and Carlson 2006).

This means that low omega-3 DHA results in lower connectivity in the brain. This knowledge brings hope that dietary alterations can potentially act as a preventative measure.

Globally, researchers are on a quest to find novel ways to treat, cure and even prevent brain disorders such as Alzheimer's disease, epilepsy and traumatic brain injury. When thinking about how to protect our brains, we should consider the composition of the brain and feeding it the fuel it is made up of – essential fatty acids and, of course, water. One of my goals is to advocate for research and awareness into the therapeutic role of nutrition in mental health and neurodevelopmental differences. There will be more information on DHA in Chapter 5, but if you wish to start increasing the omega-3s in your family's diet now, you can look at the end of the book for recipes, many of which include seafood which is rich in omega-3s.

Chapter Takeaway

- **ADHD often has other disorders overlapping with it.**
- **There are records of ADHD going back to the late 18th century.**
- **Neuroimaging research has allowed us to see that there are differences in brain function and, in some cases, the structure of the brain between individuals with and without ADHD.**
- **Low omega-3 levels have been found in people with ADHD and can be corrected by eating fish and seafood or by taking supplements.**

TAKE A STEP

Increase your family's seafood and fish intake by using some of the recipes given at the end of this book.

Chapter 2

The Gut–Brain Axis

In this chapter I describe the connection between the brain and the gut (stomach), and how the health of one affects the other. The environment of the gut can have effects on learning, memory, mood and stress responses – all factors in ADHD symptoms. Gastrointestinal issues are more common in people who experience poor mental health. Learning how food can affect the brain will help you make conscious and more deliberate choices about how you feed your own and, even more importantly perhaps, a growing child's brain.

The way to the brain is through the stomach. I know that's not the saying, but it really does apply. The fact is, our grey matter and our guts are linked in ways we could barely have guessed a couple of decades ago. In fact, we now know that a high percentage of the chemical required for our happiness – serotonin – is actually made in the gut and then transported via a special route called the vagus nerve directly into our brain. Hence the gut is often referred to as our 'second brain'.

There is now a significant body of research demonstrating that our psychological profile and brain function are engaged in an intimate relationship with the gut. Although this interaction, commonly referred to as the the 'gut–brain axis', has been recognized for decades, it's only during the past 10 years that new evidence has shown how this two-way relationship works (Cryan and O'Mahony 2011). This evidence has huge implications for brain conditions such as ADHD and ASD, as well as our quest to eat our way to good brain health.

Gut bacteria – also referred to collectively as the gut microbiome – directly shape who we are, impacting our learning, memory, mood and stress response, not to mention appetite. There are also strong links between psychiatric disorders and problems with the gut. The collective research in this field has increased our knowledge and understanding of the trillions of bacteria that make their home in the human gut (McVey Neufeld *et al.* 2016).

Institute for Food, Brain and Behaviour (IFBB) Charitable Trust[1]

We are what we eat. And we're simply not eating enough of the right foods to keep our brains healthy. It's a crisis of our own making – and it's getting worse. Most people know that our diet affects our physical wellbeing. But there's not enough education about the need to nourish the development and maintenance of a healthy brain. Our brains influence and dictate our intelligence, our instincts, our alertness and every aspect of our behaviour. Without the right care, all these will suffer. We need to eat less junk and more foods rich in the right micronutrients and essential fatty acids. If we don't, then our brains will not function

1 www.thinkthroughnutrition.org

properly, leading to major mental health problems and behavioural issues.

The Institute for Food Brain and Behaviour (IFBB) is a ground-breaking UK charity that aims to improve public knowledge of this link between nutrition and behaviour. We bring together scientists, nutritionists, teachers, cooks and caterers to spread our message. We target our work in four key areas: Nutrition and Mental Health, Nutrition in Education and Learning, Nutrition and Offending Behaviours, and Nutrition and the Ageing Brain.

It is generally accepted that what we eat affects our bodies, both in the short term and over months or years. It is not only reasonable but also imperative, therefore, to understand that diet also affects brain function and cognition, especially while the brain is still maturing. In extreme cases, we know that dietary changes can affect the brain in a more obvious way, over both short and long timescales. For example, very low blood sugar levels (hypoglycaemia) can distort thinking, make a person nervous or aggressive, cause them to faint, or send them into a coma. In the Netherlands and China, studies of children born during or just after famines have found that their mothers' exposure to starvation is linked to a higher risk in the child – years later – of psychiatric disorders, such as schizophrenia.

What of less extreme situations than famine? The research evidence strongly suggests that good nutrition is important not only for healthy growth, but for healthy brain function and cognition too. This is a matter of global importance. Although it may be particularly relevant to the poorest countries, even in such wealthy nations as the UK poverty is a major risk factor for poor nutrition, with consequences for children's health and development. A large-scale study of UK children, for example, found that high consumption of junk food at age four-and-a-half was associated with significantly more hyperactivity at age seven.

ADHD is a major contributor to poor educational outcomes, typically treated by powerful psychoactive drugs such as Ritalin. To the extent that a better diet does reduce levels of hyperactivity in schools, acting on that knowledge is likely to improve both children's health – by sparing them drug treatment – and their learning outcomes.

The science at present is enough to suggest that diet may have a considerable impact not only on children's bodies, but also on their ability to learn and to handle the attentional and behavioural demands of a modern school environment. Given the highly competitive, exam-driven nature of both schools and the workplace thereafter, children need all the help they can get to succeed. Compared with the other ways our society deals with educational failure, dietary interventions are cheap and simple and are unlikely to have adverse side effects. If they can assist with learning, be it only by enabling the child to focus on work for longer, they must be worth considering.

High dietary consumption of the omega-3s found in fish oils in early life may have long-lasting positive effects on cognition. Fatty acid and multivitamin supplements have repeatedly been found to improve attentional and behavioural problems in school children, as well as illness and attendance rates.

The IFBB coordinated a research trial in the Robert Clack School, Dagenham, which serves a very deprived community. We tested the effects of vitamin, mineral and omega-3 supplementation on behaviour in 13- to 16-year-olds; 196 children volunteered for the 12-week trial. One group was given the nutritional supplements while the other was given placebos. Blood samples were taken to measure the change in omega-3, omega-6, vitamin and mineral levels over the study. These were very low at the start and significantly improved in the group receiving the nutrient supplements during the study.

Although this was a small-scale trial, the results warrant serious attention. Behaviour change was measured using the Conners scale and school disciplinary records. On the disruptive behaviour scale, the students receiving the supplements improved significantly, while the pupils receiving the placebos worsened, as usually happens as the term progresses. The behaviour of the worst improved more than that of the best-behaving teenagers while they took the nutrient supplements. These results suggest that nutritional supplementation can significantly improve behaviour in disadvantaged school children. This study is just one piece of a large body of evidence with similar results.

Dr Jonathan Tammam, principal researcher on the Robert Clack School study and IFBB fellow, said, 'Our research adds to the growing body of evidence that nutrition can impact on the cognitive health and behaviour of children, not least from underprivileged backgrounds. These findings have implications for public health policy and are useful in working towards our aim of understanding how improvements in dietary intake can benefit the health and lives of individuals and society.'

It is our responsibility to take such science forward into the lives of these individuals, to the benefit of all.

A healthy gut and brain is connected to gut bacteria. Bacteria existed on this planet more than one-and-a-half billion years before mammals. They have co-existed with us from the very beginning, occupying many different ecological niches on and in our bodies. In some cases, these bacteria are simply opportunistic stowaways that do neither good nor harm. In other cases, these bacteria can bloom and produce toxins that may be harmful to the host. For the most part, however, the relationship is mutually beneficial in that we provide a nutrient-rich and protected habitat while these bacteria break down otherwise indigestible foods and provide us with previously inaccessible nutrients. It is estimated that the average mass of microorganisms living in an adult human intestine is approximately 1–2kg. In a healthy human being there is a core microbiota (group of microorganisms or bacteria) that features around 17 different bacterial groups central to our health (Falony *et al.* 2016).

Certain genes involved in the formation of neurons in the brain are similar to those in the gastrointestinal tract. The composition of an individual's gut microbiota depends on many factors, including:

- Mode of delivery at birth (i.e. by Caesarean section or vaginal delivery).
- Genetic inheritance and predisposition.
- Location at birth (i.e. home or hospital).
- Source of nutrition (breast milk or formula fed).
- Antibiotic exposure of mother or infant.
- Levels of hygiene in the hospital and at home.

Once the baby is weaned to complementary foods and multiple sources of dietary fibre, the microbiome undergoes a dramatic change and begins to assume the composition of the adult gut. From that time on, environmental factors such as nutrition, stress exposure, physical exercise, exposure to infections and other diseases also contribute to the balance. The previously held notion that an unborn child is exposed to a germ-free environment during pregnancy has been pretty much blown out of the water (Lurie, Lurie and Children's Hospital of Chicago 2019). It is also currently understood that initial colonization of the gut occurs during the birth process through a faecal–oral transfer of the mother's gut bacteria to the infant. This initial seeding of the baby's gut is then expanded into an infant microbiome dominated by a single species, *Bifidobacteria longum infantis*, whose growth is supported by its unique ability to utilize human milk (Funkhouser and Bordenstein 2013).

Professor Michael Crawford, Imperial College London

Mental illness is now the greatest burden of ill health, costing more than cancer and heart disease combined (Trautmann, Rehm and Wittchen 2016).

In my opinion, it has gained this notoriety because people were not interested in the brain and were even less interested in the fact that the nutrition of the brain and body are served by different sets of nutrients. Protein is the buzzword of expert food committees and TV adverts. Protein is genuinely a determinant of body growth. However, we all know just by looking at it that the brain is a fatty organ. It requires special fatty acids. The omega-3 docosahexaenoic acid (DHA) is a key signalling molecule, but is scarce in the standard Western diet.

The source of DHA is primarily the marine food web, so it is not surprising to reflect that the brain evolved in the sea. When dinosaurs evolved on land they gained massive body sizes but had tiny brains, so much so that their spinal cords had to have signal booster systems.

When the mammals arrived, they had smaller bodies and bigger brains. They were smarter than the giant dinosaurs before them, and a significant proportion went back into the sea where they had access to the marine food web, back where the brain first evolved. That gave them even bigger brains. Take a zebra, for example. It has a brain size of about 350g. Take a marine mammal of similar body size – a dolphin, which has a 1.7kg brain! This information is well known. Its implication is, however, ignored. We have behaved like the people who could not see the wood for the trees.

During the Second World War, fish and seafood were not rationed. Every mother and pregnant woman was given cod liver oil, milk and orange juice free, delivered to her front door by the milkman! After the war the game was 'PRODUCTION'. Research centres for animal and crop production were set up. The aim was fast weight gain, and protein was good for body growth. What went wrong was that while this was fine for cows, sheep, pigs, cats and dogs, it was not so good for *H. sapiens*, where the brain is the priority.

I like to get my messages from physiology rather than expert committees. The expert committees have been emphasizing protein quality for over half a century. They were wrong. All they had to do was recognize that the priority of *H. sapiens* happened to be the *sapiens* bit. So, what is the message from physiology? The composition of human milk sums it up: it has the least protein of all the large mammals, but is rich in the essential fats needed for finishing off brain growth after birth.

So how exactly does the gut influence brain function, and in particular, why do children with neurodevelopmental conditions such as ASD and ADHD seem to be particularly sensitive to and affected by gut health?

Recent studies show that between 30 and 50 per cent of individuals with ASD manifest ADHD symptoms (in particular, at pre-school age), and correspondingly, it is estimated that at least two-thirds of individuals with ADHD display features of ASD (Davis and Kollins 2012). Because of this, there is much overlap in research as well. In a 2015 study, children were supplemented with either friendly bacteria called *Lactobacillus rhamnosus GG* (ATCC 53103) or a placebo during their first six months of life and then checked over the next 13 years. The results showed that those children with a diagnosis of ASD or ADHD had lower levels of *Bifidobacteria* species (the predominant bacteria in an infant's gut) than babies and children without a diagnosis. Specifically, ADHD or ASD was diagnosed in 6 out of 35 (17.1%) of children in the placebo group and none in the probiotic group ($n = 40$) by the age of 13. The authors concluded that probiotic supplementation early in life may reduce the risk of the development of ADHD and ASD symptoms later in childhood, possibly via mechanisms related to gut microbiota composition (Partty *et al.* 2015).

You've probably seen the words 'probiotic' and 'prebiotic' on various 'healthy' food items in the supermarket, such as yoghurts. You've probably wondered whether they're important. They are! Prebiotics are indigestible foods mainly in the form of carbohydrates (fibre), which selectively promote the growth of specific gut bacteria and provide indirect health benefits to the host, while probiotics are live bacteria that only transiently inhabit the gut. The role of gut microbiota in psychiatric illnesses, and in particular, emotional and physiological stress, has captured both public and scientific interest. Recent research has demonstrated that changes in neurotransmitters *in the intestine* can lead to changes in behaviour, including the development of mood disorders. This two-way relationship takes place across hormonal, immunological and neural pathways. This, then, is the amazing reality of the 'gut–brain axis'.

Below I outline some of the research studies that make these connections.

Several studies have shown beneficial changes in gut microbiota composition as a result of omega-3 supplementation (Ghosh *et al.* 2013; Kaliannan *et al.* 2015; Yu *et al.* 2014), whereas, on the other hand, diets rich in omega-6 can cause disruption to gut microbiota (Ghosh *et al.* 2013). Young people, more than ever before, are exposed to a wide range of unhealthy food options resulting in a surfeit of pro-inflammatory omega-6 and simultaneous decrease in the healthy and essential omega-3 fats. Add to this reductions in fibre and excessive sugar and you have a cocktail that can markedly alter the composition of the gut microbiome and lead to brain dysfunction, behavioural problems such as aggression and violence, and psychiatric illness (Bruce-Keller *et al.* 2015; Cordain *et al.* 2005; Eaton and Eaton 2000; Hibbeln 2007; Hibbeln, Nieminen and Lands 2004).

One of the first studies to suggest an association between autoimmune dysfunction, low omega-3 status and hyperactivity was published by Colquhoun and Bunday in 1981. They surveyed the diets of 214 children (161 of them boys) who attended the Hyperactive Children's Support Group (HACSG) in London, and reported that boys with ADHD-type symptoms had fatty acid deficiency. For example, they reported that two-thirds of the children suffered from polydipsia (excessive thirst), had zinc values below the normal range, and suffered from allergies including eczema and asthma, with intolerances to milk and wheat – all of which are symptoms directly or indirectly related to fatty acid deficiency (Colquhoun and Bunday 1981). Although this study was not a clinical trial, it was published as a medical hypothesis and led to the closer investigation by other researchers globally into the potential link between food allergies, omega-3 polyunsaturated fatty acids (PUFAs) deficiency and hyperactive behaviour.

Other nutrients known to positively alter gut microbiota include polyphenols. These are compounds that occur naturally in plants, vegetables (e.g. artichokes, olives, carrots, celery), fruits (e.g. blueberries, strawberries, raspberries), certain fruits juices (e.g. grape juice), rye bread and dark chocolate.

What to Do Next

In a nutshell, nutrition plays a critical role in both neurodevelopment and the establishment of healthy gut microbiota. And that's because the two are linked. The microbiota are crucial for vitamin absorption and food digestion. Changes in its composition take place over the course of child development and continue with age, which is why it's never too early or too late to eat well for good gut/brain health. The teenage years are thought to be a particularly vulnerable time for alterations in gut microbiota, which can be caused by specific environmental stressors including sleep disturbance and exposure to drugs, alcohol, stress, antibiotic usage, and our old enemy, poor diet (McVey Neufeld *et al.* 2016).

So what can you do if you are a parent, or work with parents and children, to alleviate concerns you may have about a child's gut health? The first step is to seek a consultation from a trained professional such as a registered nutritionist or dietician. They will guide you and your child through the evaluation process and make a referral for laboratory tests to assess for food allergies and intolerances. This should include a stool test to assess the state of intestinal immune function, beneficial bacteria levels, intestinal health and inflammation markers. Additionally, faecal matter can reveal probiotic levels along with microbes present in the gut, both the good and the bad type.

With this information, modifications can be made, such as allergen-free diets and the introduction of gut-friendly foods. A registered nutritionist and dietician will inform you of the benefits of an adequate daily intake of omega-3 fats and eating foods rich in polyphenols and antioxidants, as well as lowering intake of omega-6 fats from processed foods such as biscuits (cookies), cakes, sweets (candy), pastries and so on. Complementary and alternative medicines that are already used in these patient groups may also help manage behavioural symptoms, including the addition of probiotics containing beneficial bacteria strains or non-digestible oligosaccharides (a specific type of carbohydrate). Probiotics can be found in fermented foods such as miso, kefir, sauerkraut, kimchi, tempeh, kombucha and yoghurt, as well as in powdered or capsule form from health food stores.

Chapter Takeaway

- **The gut and the brain share a connection called the gut–brain axis.**
- **Children with ADHD have been shown to have lower levels of omega-3s and of *Bifidobacteria* species (the predominant bacteria in an infant's gut).**
- **One study indicates that probiotic supplementation early in life may reduce the risk of the development of ADHD and ASD symptoms later in childhood.**
- **Seeing a registered nutritionist or dietician will help you determine the health of your child's gut and could guide you in how to improve their gut microbiome, thereby helping the brain through the gut–brain axis.**

TAKE A STEP

Include foods with polyphenols and probiotics in your and your family's meals, for example carrots, celery, olives, grape juice, blueberries, dark chocolate and probiotic yoghurts. Try the Tropical Fruit Salad recipe or a blended juice (see the recipes section at the end of the book).

Chapter 3

Food as Medicine and Food as Poison

> **Let food be thy medicine and medicine be thy food.**
> **Hippocrates**

Consider this: your child has just been diagnosed with ADHD. As he is only six years old you don't necessarily want to rush into medicating him. You have heard that changing his diet might help and you have admitted that his current diet is not the best. You are looking for advice about what to eat and what to avoid, and which ingredients might make life easier to manage. Where do you turn first? Not to your family medical practitioner, sadly.

Your family medical practitioner or medical care provider probably knows very little about nutrition. It's not their fault. It's just that nutrition – unlike prescription drugs – is not a compulsory part of the medical student's training. The BBC published an article in March 2018 by Sheila Dillon, a presenter on Radio 4's *Food Programme*, highlighting the concern that medical students receive little or no nutritional training. Those medical students, a few years down the line, are our family medical practitioners.

For some time now, many research studies have reported a link between low levels of vitamin D and depression. A review published by Simon Spedding (2014) re-evaluated the published literature and concluded that vitamin D was moderately favourable in the treatment of depression, with comparable effects to antidepressant medication. Yet you could almost predict that your medical practitioner will not refer you to have your vitamin D levels assessed or link the two. Instead, patients will likely be asked a series of checklist questions confirming the incidence and severity of symptoms, and will then quite likely be offered a prescription for antidepressant medication.

There is no doubt that certain medications are necessary and life saving. However, increasingly we are simply not moving beyond the prescription pad. The US, for example, represents only 5 per cent of the world's population yet consumes 75 per cent of the world's prescription medication. Psychiatric medications are not a cure but they are a band aid. They won't eliminate the underlying condition but can provide transient relief and reduce symptoms.

For ADHD, treatment is typically synonymous with psychostimulant medication (methylphenidate). However, National Institute for Health and Care Excellence (NICE) (2018) guidelines[1] recommend that medication for children aged five and over should only be prescribed if:

- their ADHD symptoms are still causing a persistent significant impairment in at least one domain after environmental modifications have been implemented and reviewed

---

1 See www.nice.org.uk/guidance/ng87/chapter/Recommendations.

- they and their parents and carers have discussed information about ADHD (see recommendation 1.5.4)
- a baseline assessment has been carried out (see recommendation 1.7.4).

Recommendation 1.7.4 also gives further guidance on medication. There is evidence for at least short-term effectiveness in around two-thirds of patients with ADHD. However, there are a number of reported adverse side effects that can include: slowing of growth, anorexia, sleep problems, irritability, headaches, abdominal pain, emergence of tics, rebound effects (i.e. when the dose wears off), and subsequent heightened ADHD symptoms such as emotional instability and depressed mood (Taylor *et al.* 2004). Similarly, non-stimulant medications for ADHD such as atomoxetine are linked with increased irritability, agitation, self-harming and suicidal behaviour, reduced appetite and weight loss, increased blood pressure and heart rate, and the rare possibility of liver damage (Taylor *et al.* 1991). It is estimated that around one-third of cases experience little benefit from medication, or discontinue use due to side effects, while some still require assistance with residual symptoms. A proportion of parents simply feel uncomfortable with the decision to give pharmacological drugs to their children and instead seek alternative or complementary interventions (Sarris *et al.* 2011).

The production of Ritalin and the legal production of amphetamine in the form of Adderall and Dexedrine in the US has soared since 1990 as a means of controlling hyperactive, impulsive or inattentive behaviour. According to the United Nations (UN), the US now produces and consumes about 85 per cent of the world's methylphenidate (the chemical name for Ritalin). However, the medication of children appears divided and in some unfortunate cases out of control, with parents losing their parental rights and facing jail for not medicating their children, while others are sent to jail for selling similar chemical compounds on the streets (Breggin

2007). In the UK, and indeed most of Europe, the prescribing of pharmacological interventions for ADHD in children is considered only in chronic cases and when all other interventions have been exhausted, although the idea that a diagnosis of ADHD is synonymous with medication is still mainstream thought.

Psychiatrists and clinicians are frequently caught up in a narrative of symptoms, diagnoses, data and the automatic prescribing of pharmacological medications, and yet, nutrition – or lack of it – fails to feature in their diagnostic assessments. Our healthcare systems may be extremely proficient at diagnosing mental illness and making subsequent pharmacological interventions, but long-term solutions and the role of prevention are not being addressed.

Medication does *not* have all the answers. If only it were that simple! There is now an abundance of evidence supporting the combination of both nutrition and exercise to slow ageing and mild cognitive decline, and improve depression, attention deficits and mood disorders. In the same way a wound needs to heal, a holistic approach is recommended to treat the brain. There is not a one-size-fits-all approach to treatment – ideally interventions should be a combination of personalized integrative care, and include dietary changes, nutritional supplements, exercise, meditation and therapy.

Dr Richard Soppitt, Consultant Child Psychiatrist, CAMHS Sussex Partnership NHS Trust

Frederick Still, a developmental paediatrician, identified children with ADHD in 1902. Over a hundred years later, we have come a very long way in understanding that ADHD is a heterogeneous group with a vast array of environmental, genetic and epigenetic factors leading to its phenotype.

ADHD has survived social constructionism, post-modernism and suspicions about 'bad pharma'. The 'both/and' discourse that allows for looking at the meaning of ADHD for a family or young person, the pros and cons of a label, and also the evidence for treatment effect sizes, have allowed for a marriage of pharmacology and family interventions. A combined approach makes the most sense, but often families do not want to feel blamed, stigmatized or disempowered by professionals. On the other hand, a narrow approach to treatment that does not see the biopsychosocial does our young people and adult sufferers a disservice. The increasing recognition in NICE guideline iterations on parenting and behavioural management recognizes the need to try non-pharmacological interventions before, during and after medication.

Most ADHD clinics I have worked in have unsung heroes – the ADHD nurses. They are often the ones who carry massive burdens of numbers, work tirelessly to mediate and advocate in the SEN system, and are struggling with fewer and fewer child psychiatrists available to diagnose and supervise their prescribing practice if they are independent non-medical prescribers. Shared care is vital with family medical practitioners as this de-stigmatizes care and provides a local engagement with families, which is essential. With austerity, shared care may be under threat, and the drive to use cheaper medications may lead to sub-optimal interventions, but hopefully we will not go back to the bad old days of Ritalin three times a day. Omega-3 has been seen as helpful in other aspects of mental health such as 'at-risk mental states'. As yet it has had only a small part in ADHD treatment, but it is unlikely we have heard the last of it.

I recall being surprised at the long-term outcomes of those with ADHD who, by the time they have reached their 30s, do not have significantly lower employment rates or higher benefit claiming rates compared with their non-ADHD counterparts (Basset-Grundy and Butler 2004). As child psychiatrists we sadly do not see the wonderful myelination and maturation processes into the 20s combined with young people taking control of their destiny and choosing paths that suit them as individuals, finding their own round holes and recovering from the process of previously being pushed into square ones. Proper youth services, that is, 16–25, would make a difference in the transitional arrangements for young people who often fall off the conveyor belt of CAMHS (Child and Adolescent Mental Health Services) or community paediatrics into confusion or lack of support. Inventive commissioning that marries CAMHS and community paediatrics better around ADHD and ASD pathways would be on my future wish list. Much valuable time is wasted moving between services and falling between stools.

For the future, it would be good to appreciate that a diagnosis of ADHD does not stipulate the causal mechanisms, and so the old chestnut of 'this child cannot have ADHD because they have experienced brain trauma or attachment disruptions, etc.' will become more balanced, and there will be recognition that all treatment modalities, including those for ADHD, can assist young people even if they have an acquired an ADHD presentation or one that arises out of early attachment difficulties.

Recognition of the impact of an ADHD inattentive subtype, and a clearer understanding of specific learning difficulties presenting as ADHD and vice versa, would be welcome. Neuroimaging diagnostics, combined family therapy and medication clinics, an acceptance that the ADHD diagnosis is not an excuse for bad parenting in the tabloids, and more SEN support for those with ADHD whose headline behaviours mean their underlying needs are not assessed will hopefully come to pass.

The educational outcomes of those with ADHD are still far too low, and the educational under-achievement perhaps more so for boys than girls indicates that the way we engage our children in learning needs to be meaningful and build on their strengths and individual learning styles. One size never fits all in education. Exercise, creativity and building self-esteem through extracurricular activities are all essential resiliency strategies for our current and future children with ADHD. Their energy, ability to multitask and related talent for humour could, of course, lead to the same discussion we are having with ASD and neurodiversity.

It may be that ADHD is just another term for being unique, walking a road less travelled, and we had better recognize the strengths and quirkiness of the children and strive to help them be themselves while protecting them from the worst aspects of society's 'one size fits all' dogma. Of course, where there is significant impairment we can assist and remediate the environment, including addressing sensory processing with skilled occupational therapists, and where necessary the neurochemistry, to add quality to their lives.

Most parents, teachers and indeed policy-makers understand that nutrition is important for physical health, to prevent obesity and early onset diabetes in childhood, and to safeguard against cardiovascular disease and cancer in later life. However, the importance of nutrition for brain health and optimal function is almost completely overlooked, even in the 21st century. This is despite public predictions from the World Health Organization (WHO) of a 50 per cent increase in child mental illness by 2020. In terms of schooling, one in four children in every classroom have a learning and/or behavioural difference, while prescriptions for psychostimulant medications have increased almost threefold in the last decade as a means of controlling hyperactive, impulsive and inattentive symptoms.

A Word about Self-Medicating and Addiction

Unfortunately, a proportion of the population, especially those with poor mental health and diagnostic conditions such as ADHD, will succumb to the art of *self-medicating* with nicotine, alcohol, cannabis, cocaine or prescription pills such as Adderall or Xanax as a way of coping with underlying depression, anxiety, undiagnosed ADHD, or all of the above. Several research studies have confirmed that those with undiagnosed ADHD have an increased risk of the development of substance use disorders (SUD) as well as a tendency towards binge eating with sugary, processed junk food. Self-medicating is a known phenomenon in teenagers and adults with ADHD, and the risks are thought to be increased in children not taking prescribed medication (Biederman 1995; Wilens *et al.* 2003). The fact is that young people with ADHD are wired to be impulsive and risk-taking; they also gravitate to novelty and can be sensation-seeking. The experimental taking of substances is common during the teenage years, but use is greater in ADHD, starting with alcohol, nicotine and marijuana, and can progress rapidly to other drugs including MDMA (ecstasy), ketamine, Xanax, synthetic highs, cocaine and methamphetamines.

Essentially, some of these substances can temporarily calm symptoms of ADHD – for example, alcohol can settle internal restlessness and suppress busy brains. However, over time, habitual use will damage cellular activity, and can lead to increased symptoms of depression and anxiety and significantly reduce brain activity, as shown in MRI or PET (positron emission tomography) scans (Amen 2013).

Tobacco use is higher in individuals with ADHD by approximately double compared to non-diagnosed controls (Wilens 2004).

Furthermore, it is associated with an earlier onset of smoking, higher rates of use and greater difficulty with abstinence (Wilens *et al.* 2008). Both nicotine and traditional pharmacological medications for ADHD operate as stimulants or 'uppers'. This shared functionality is consistent with the hypothesis that nicotine is used as a type of self-medication in these patient groups (Conners *et al.* 1996; Levin *et al.* 1996). The temporary effects of nicotine have been documented to enhance memory, reduce anxiety and tension, and improve symptoms of impulsivity, alertness, concentration and attention in adults with ADHD, all of which are considered to play a reinforcing role in the relationship between ADHD and smoking. Reducing the symptoms of ADHD by using medication (e.g. Ritalin) impacts the dopamine active transporter (DAT) and has been found to significantly delay the onset of smoking in young adults (Dougherty *et al.* 1999; Monuteaux *et al.* 2008).

An estimated 50 per cent of adults with ADHD have substance abuse issues, and this is likely to be an unconscious effort to normalize their own brain function. Teenage boys will often tell me that smoking cannabis 'makes them feel normal' but it is the after-effects that do the damage – mood swings, decreased motivation, depression and anxiety.

Substance use is a way of self-regulating or normalizing the dopamine-production function. The neurotransmitter dopamine is linked to feelings of pleasure, reward, motivation and mood. Although the effects are only transient, we have learned how to manipulate our brain's pleasure centres, and that keeps us coming back for more. If a laboratory animal is given the choice of alcohol or water, they will persistently return for alcohol, and so dependence begins very quickly. The same is true for cocaine and sugar. Introduce electric shocks to the lab rat prior to obtaining the chemical hit and they will persist regardless (Yap and Miczek 2009). This is the nature of the process of addiction.

Self-medicating in the long term does not work and only leads to heightened symptoms, the development of physical and psychological addictions and burnout. All brains are wired to seek pleasure and avoid pain. Substances such as nicotine, alcohol, cocaine and sugar all provide a chemically induced hit of dopamine, resulting in pleasure. No wonder they are addictive – they make people feel euphoric!

The habitual consumption of unhealthy foods, alcohol and substances upsets the biochemistry of the brain, placing it in a chronic pro-inflammatory state that increases vulnerability for addictions, neurodegeneration (i.e. degeneration of the nervous system, especially brain neurons) and psychiatric disease. There is a significant role for nutrition in prevention and disease management in non-communicative diseases, and ultimately in restoring and maintaining brain health.

Bad Food/Good Food

The human body is remarkable, with healing abilities like no other known entity. Arguably Mother Nature provides all we need for a healthy body; however, the dramatic change in food manufacturing in favour of mass food production, profit and shelf life has compromised this. Sick people often get sicker, and this is quite simply in my mind because many of the 50,000 commercially available supermarket foods (Malito 2017) can arguably be hazardous, affecting the ability of our bodily cells to function as they are programmed to and serving as catalysts for disease development. The habitual consumption of refined foods and sugars is wreaking havoc with our physical and mental health, and while many of us recognize unhealthy foods are bad for our bodies, the effects on brain function are often overlooked. This is especially relevant for mental health, and in particular for the symptom management of mood disorders.

A worldwide consortium released a statement, published in 2015 in *The Lancet* (a leading scientific journal), advocating for nutritional science to be mainstream in psychiatry:

> The emerging and compelling evidence for nutrition as a crucial factor in the high prevalence and incidence of mental disorders suggests that diet is as important to psychiatry as it is cardiology, endocrinology, and gastroenterology. (Sarris *et al.* 2015)

Collectively, we need a fundamental change in thinking to recognize that certain foods can act in comparable ways to medications. Evidence-based educational and medical training are necessary to bring this about, and, of course, a shift in attitude to approach mental health from multiple perspectives, using a personalized, evidence-based approach beyond just the prescription pad. Many studies have demonstrated that changing nutritional habits can help improve our overall brain health, reduce inflammatory markers in our brain that can lead to depression and other mental health issues, and positively impact wellbeing and mood. One of the key barriers preventing the application of this knowledge is the fact that medical students and those already trained as clinicians and psychiatrists are given or have received very little nutritional training.

Robert K. McNamara, Department of Psychiatry and Behavioral Neuroscience, University of Cincinnati College of Medicine, and Francisco Romo-Nava, Lindner Center of HOPE

Nutrition in Psychiatric Practice: A Promising but Neglected Alliance

Psychiatric disorders including ADHD are typically chronic or recurring illnesses associated with significant psychosocial disability. The initial onset of ADHD frequently occurs during early childhood, and symptoms commonly persist into adulthood. Childhood development is associated with rapid maturational changes in the prefrontal cortex, and imaging studies indicate that ADHD is associated with structural and functional abnormalities in the prefrontal cortex.

First-line treatments for ADHD are typically cognitive behavioural therapy or psychostimulant medications including methylphenidate or amphetamine. Although stimulant medications are effective for reducing ADHD symptoms, long-term treatment may lead to adverse side effects, including sleep problems, growth retardation and elevated aggression in the case of amphetamine-type drugs. However, treatment discontinuation frequently precipitates symptom relapse, suggesting these medications do not correct the underlying neuropathological mechanism.

Other medications routinely used in psychiatric practice, including antidepressants, mood stabilizers and antipsychotics, also frequently lead to adverse side effects with long-term use, and symptom relapse commonly occurs following treatment discontinuation. Therefore, available pharmacological medicines are suboptimal, and alternative or complementary treatments are needed to improve long-term outcomes for patients.

Over the past few decades there has been growing interest in the potential role of diet and nutrition in the pathophysiology and treatment of psychiatric disorders. Evidence from cross-sectional studies and meta-analyses suggests that ADHD may be associated with a constellation of micronutrient deficiencies, including vitamin D, zinc, iron, magnesium, manganese and essential fatty acids. Although currently controversial, overconsumption of processed sugar, synthetic food colouring and preservatives, and hyper-allergenic foods may be associated with attention problems, hyperactivity and aggression in children and adolescents.

Controlled intervention trials suggest that dietary

supplementation with broad-spectrum micronutrients (vitamins and minerals), or long-chain omega-3 fatty acids, or a restricted elimination diet, can reduce cognitive and emotional symptoms in ADHD patients. It is also notable that prospective longitudinal studies suggest that maternal deficiencies in micronutrients, including vitamin D and long-chain omega-3 fatty acids, may also increase the risk for developing ADHD in their offspring.

A growing body of evidence from animal developmental studies further suggest that micronutrient deficiencies can negatively impact brain development and function in a manner that is relevant to ADHD. For example, developmental omega-3 fatty acid deficiency is associated with an enduring impairment in dopamine neurotransmission. Taken collectively, this body of evidence provides an empirical foundation supporting a potential role of diet and nutrition in the aetiology and progression of ADHD.

Although diet and nutrition are slowly gaining momentum in psychiatric research, they remain a largely neglected component of psychiatric practice. This is not unique to psychiatry, and many other fields of medicine, including those more closely associated with nutrition-related diseases such as cardiovascular disease, rarely consult with their patients about diet and nutrition (Kahan and Manson 2017). This has been attributed to several factors, including limited physician training in nutrition and a general lack of coordination between the two fields. There are also practical constraints, including a lack of time to address diet during a patient visit, as well as challenges associated with the implementation of dietary modifications, including non-compliance and costs associated with dietary supplements or more nutritious foods.

Nevertheless, there is emerging consensus that nutritional counselling and nutritional medicine become incorporated into routine psychiatric practice (Sarris *et al.* 2015). Such an alliance would be particularly valuable within the context of a 'clinical staging' model, in which safer and better-tolerated interventions could be used in the earlier stages of illness followed by more aggressive treatments that may pose greater health risks for non-responsive cases. For example, this could entail documentation and evaluation of the patient's habitual diet and performing blood tests to screen for food hypersensitivities and micronutrient deficiencies, followed by targeted dietary supplementation or systematic diet modifications. This approach would either rule in or rule out a dietary component. If such measures do not satisfactorily reduce symptoms over time, conventional treatments could then be initiated as required.

The role of nutrition in human disease is not a new concept, and many historical precedents exist for a causal relationship between chronic micronutrient deficiency and adverse physical and/or neurological symptoms. Notable examples include vitamin C (ascorbic acid) deficiency leading to scurvy, vitamin A deficiency leading to night blindness, and vitamin B (niacin) deficiency leading to pellagra, which is associated with psychiatric symptoms. These single-nutrient deficiencies serve to remind us of the critical role they play in human health, and emphasize the potential impact of multiple nutrient deficiencies on normal brain development and their role in neurodevelopmental disorders, including ADHD.

Ultimately, the incorporation of nutrition into routine psychiatric practice will provide an alternative to the standard pharmaceutical approach, and therefore the opportunity to tailor and optimize treatment for patients. Such an alliance is currently feasible and warranted.

I recently visited a community mental health drop-in centre in South West London. I was shown around and introduced to the services the centre offered. There were therapy rooms for people with serious mental health conditions such as schizophrenia and bipolar, in addition to those suffering with addictions and anxiety. I was told by one of the workers that they provided free food and warm drinks, and given it was a cold winter's night and the centre was pretty busy, I could see great benefits to this.

Then I was taken to the kitchen and looked at some of the food laid out on the table. I saw pastries, sausage rolls, crisps and other processed foods – apparently free donations (leftovers) from a well-known local bakery. The coffee machine was very popular, too, I was told. I could imagine! Although delighted that visitors to the centre were receiving hot and, importantly, free food, my heart sank at the absence of any healthy food options.

Most people are unaware of the consequences to brain health if they are *not* eating the *right* foods. They may even have no idea that their physical bodies might be nutritionally impoverished and that nutritional insufficiencies can critically alter the way their brains function, influencing mood, attention, behaviour and critically, the ability to learn. This applies to everyone, even those without ADHD.

The effects of food additives on children's hyperactive behaviour were investigated in a randomized, placebo-controlled clinical trial in 2007 (McCann *et al.* 2007). This trial recruited 153 three-year-olds and 144 eight/nine-year-olds. The children were randomly assigned to one of three drinks: two contained artificial food colours and additives (AFCA, for short) including sodium benzoate (a preservative), and the other was a placebo drink. The trial measured hyperactivity based on observed behaviours and ratings by teachers and parents, along with a computerized attention span test for the eight/nine-year-old group. The results demonstrated that artificial colours or a sodium benzoate preservative (or both) had a significant adverse effect for all the age groups when compared against the placebo group (McCann *et al.* 2007). Many of the behavioural reactions resembled symptoms one would expect to observe in a child diagnosed with ADHD. In other words, the AFCA drinks increased hyperactive behaviours, that is, inattention, impulsivity and over-activity in children. As hyperactivity is also associated with overall educational difficulties including reading abilities, it is safe to say that foods containing these artificial additives should be avoided. Especially during school time!

Research in this area is nothing new. In 1975, Dr Benjamin Feingold found that removing exposure to food additives resulted in up to half of children with ADHD returning to normal behaviour when key synthetic colours and flavours were removed from their diets (Feingold 1975). This study was replicated in 1976, with the researchers hoping to disprove the earlier findings, only to find their results reinforcing Feingold's evidence (Conners *et al.* 1976).

Chemical additives in processed foods make our brain cells vulnerable to damage and even cell death. Despite this knowledge there are over 12,000 detectible neurotoxic substances in commonly consumed foods and drinks. Neurotoxins are substances that hamper the electrical activity of nerve cells and prevent them from working properly. The toxins interact with neurons either by overstimulating them, resulting in cell death, or by interrupting their communication processes. Neurotoxins are not regulated by the US Food and Drug Administration (FDA) or the European Food Standards Agency (EFSA), and it is children who are the most vulnerable, as their brains undergo major stages of development as they grow.

Food manufacturers have cleverly distorted Mother Nature's foods and replaced them with processed foods with laundry lists of 35 ingredients or more. This is most evident in breakfast cereals. Let's take the popular Lucky Charms as an example:

> Whole grain oats, sugar, oat flour, corn syrup, corn starch, salt, trisodium phosphate, colour added, natural and artificial flavour,

> vitamin E (mixed tocopherois), confectionery coating: sugar, palm kernel oil, maltodextrin, yogurt powder: cultured non-fat milk, whey protein concentrate, yogurt cultures, non-fat milk, soy lecithin, natural flavour, marshmallows (sugar, modified corn starch, corn syrup, dextrose, gelatin, calcium carbonate, coloured with yellow 5&6, blue 1, red 40, artificial flavour), crisp rice (rice flour, barley malt extract, salt), rapeseed (canola) oil, fructose, high-fructose corn syrup, sugar. Contains 2% or less of: glycerin, maltodextrin, sorbitol, water, gelatin, salt, artificial flavour.

This cereal is 37 per cent sugar by weight. With the exception of whole grain oats, these ingredients have little nutritional benefit. In fact, most are artificial. Take just two of these food-type substances as an example: yellow 6 is linked to hyperactivity and banned in most European countries, whereas high-fructose corn syrup (HFCS) is a type of industrialized sweetener found in countless food products that can elevate triglycerides levels (a type of fat), which are linked to the development of a dangerous medical condition called metabolic syndrome. Furthermore, HFCS is metabolized differently to the fructose found naturally in fruit, which also contain beneficial soluble fibre. These artificial sweeteners can alter healthy gut flora and promote weight gain, leading to obesity. Are these really the type of foods we should be feeding our children?

I recommend inspecting food labels and avoiding food items that go to great lengths to convince you they are healthy, such as 'fat-free' or 'extra light' or 'heart-healthy', as chances are they are not. Quite simply they are not real food, but chemically induced substitutes. We need food in order to thrive, not just survive, and we're not going to thrive on a cocktail of preservatives, sweeteners and flavour-enhancers.

We are finally waking up to the neurotoxic effects of common chemical compounds present in the human environment, including supermarket foods, water supplies and other household goods. Many of these have been linked to lower intellect, hyperactivity and cognitive and attention deficits. During their different developmental stages, children and adolescents are particularly vulnerable to stressors in the environment. There are many of these, including pollution, poor nutrition, family stress, economic poverty, a significant loss or separation from a loved one, emotional trauma or abuse. Increasing young people's resilience to environmental assaults by boosting their immune system and brain health is a powerful and reachable goal.

Lauren Gale, Nutritionist and Ambassador of Nutritious Minds

As well as being a qualified nutritionist I am the mother of two boys with SEN. My biggest bugbear to date has to be why so many of these children slip through the net, and although every school has a SEN department, very little, if anything, seems to get done. There are not enough resources and there is a lack of funding. I have been lucky to be in the position to move my boys out of mainstream education in the mornings and get the help they so desperately need, and I am so aware that this is very unusual and has come at a financial cost. It seems that if you are a square peg in the education system, you are going to struggle.

The other thing I have faced is the fact that SEN children in mainstream schools may not only get left behind, but on top of this, they risk never getting picked to do anything to show who they are and to build their confidence. It deeply saddens me when I go to school plays and assemblies and it is always the same children getting picked time and time again, while the SEN kids are left on the outskirts looking in at their peers getting all the approval and attention. It seems as if they just have to look on at the other children being told how wonderful they are and how they are going to go on and achieve wonderful things in their lives. This is something I experienced recently at my son's end of term leavers party. My mouth was left open and my eyes were stinging at what I felt was a blatant misunderstanding of what children with learning difficulties have to offer, which, in my opinion, is, in fact, often far more than non-SEN children. I have voiced my concerns to the school and they have promised me that they will address this situation. Life is hard enough, and this nonsense about everything being perfect has to stop; I believe it is even fuelling the current mental health crisis.

I also have Dyslexia and school didn't really work for me as I believed (wrongly) that I was *thick* as I couldn't get to grips with reading and my spelling was atrocious. As an adult, I regained the confidence to study again and I am now a nutritional therapist. I would like to say hats off to us parents who are slightly on the spectrum and bring our quirky but highly functioning brains into the workplace. This alone is inspiration for our beautiful younger generation to follow in our footsteps.

Nutrition is *not* a miracle cure and there are always other factors at play when evaluating your child's behaviour. However, it is the single most instantaneously modifiable factor – when you know your numbers! Unfortunately, your child's nutrient levels are not going to be measured by your family medical practitioner, and until this changes, they can only be investigated by seeking nutritional help from trained experts.

I am not surprised that I have observed multiple nutrient insufficiencies in the children I have worked with and tested. Vitamins, minerals and omega-3 essential fatty acids are all brain-essential, and I've seen a significant lack in children with ADHD. What I am intrigued by is why these patterns are so persistent. Much more research is needed to investigate these links. Of course, it is impossible to say exactly when these nutrients became insufficient, or whether the insufficiency has been present only recently or over a period of years. Perhaps they simply reflect dietary intake, or quite possibly there is an interplay between gut and brain health, which is less obvious. What is clear is that making nutritional changes such as increasing your intake of omega-3 fats (which also help regulate dopamine), micronutrients and vitamins can help improve brain biochemistry and reduce inflammation.

Food scientists studying the origin of disease patterns among populations know that the groups of people eating a Mediterranean diet (e.g. olive oil, nuts, seeds, green leafy vegetables, salads, fish and lean meat) not only live longer but also have lower rates of many diseases as well as lower rates of mental illness. Lean, wild meat and vegetables are the diets of our ancestors and are what we should turn to when we turn away from the typical toxic offerings. The solution is in the kitchen and going back to basics – healthy meals prepared from scratch with fresh, organic produce. I now provide two lists: 'What to include' and 'What to avoid'. Consider this a starter kit for a healthier family all around!

What to include:

- Mineral or filtered water.
- Unrefined oils such as organic extra virgin olive oil, avocado oil, macadamia nut oil.
- Balsamic or apple cider vinegar.
- Sustainably caught wild salmon, rainbow trout, mackerel, sardines, pilchards, anchovies.
- Sustainably caught white fish such as sea bass, red snapper, Dover sole, tilapia.

- Seafood (unsulfured) such as scallops, shrimp, oyster, crab, lobster, mussels.
- Green tea and other herbal hibiscus tea, organic if possible.
- Herbs, spices and garlic (chilli pepper, ginger, cinnamon, turmeric, saffron, parsley, sage, rosemary, cayenne pepper, basil, cumin, thyme, curcumin).
- Himalayan pink salt or unrefined sea salt (used sparingly).
- Nuts (pistachios, almonds, cashew, walnuts, hazelnuts, pine nuts).
- Seeds (sunflowers, chia, flax, hemp).
- Butter or ghee from grass-fed cows.
- Fresh, organic, seasonal vegetables.
- Sea vegetables (kelp, algae, seaweed).
- Fresh organic low-glycaemic fruit (avocado, tomatoes, cherries, peaches).
- Organic meat from pasture-raised, free-roaming lambs or cows.
- Organic eggs from pasture-raised, cage-free chickens.
- Complex carbohydrates and starchy vegetables such as sweet potato, squash, pumpkin.
- Whole grain such as oats, quinoa, buckwheat, millet, brown rice, spelt pasta.
- Organic wild berries (blueberries, raspberries, acai, cranberries, goji).
- Organic, unsweetened yoghurt or kefir (or goat/sheep or coconut alternatives).
- Green leaves (rocket (arugula), kale, spinach).

- Dark chocolate, above 70% cacao.
- Unrefined raw honey or maple syrup.
- A good-quality multivitamin containing B, C, D vitamins, zinc, magnesium.
- Sources of resveratrol (blueberries, raspberries, grapes), green tea extract (be careful of high caffeine content and choose caffeine-free, especially for children, due to risk of adverse side effects), blueberry extract (rich source of antioxidants with anti-inflammatory effects) and coenzyme Q10 (a heart-healthy, cell protective antioxidant found in cold water fish or supplements).

What to avoid:

- Convenience foods: make meals from scratch, using fresh, organic produce.
- White refined salt, and other artificial seasoning.
- Shop-bought sauces and dressings: make your own.
- White refined sugar, along with artificial sweeteners and other sugar replacement alternatives.
- White refined flours and produce containing these; wholemeal products are much healthier.
- Refined vegetable oils high in omega-6 fatty acids (e.g. soybean oil) and margarine containing hydrogenated vegetable oil.
- Factory-farmed meat: welfare issues apart, these contain hormones, including growth-promoting hormones, and antibiotics.
- Excess poor-quality industrially produced red meat: reduce your intake in favour of lean meat and fish.

- Processed meats as sandwich fillers, and pork containing nitrates (this includes many hams and salamis).
- Produce grown with pesticides and herbicides.
- Genetically modified organisms (GMOs).
- Foods containing high-fructose corn syrup (HFCS).
- Foods that promote calorie counting; it's the *nutritional* content that matters, not the calories (unless you have a diagnosed medical condition).
- Factory-farmed dairy products: reduce your intake, and eliminate them altogether if possible.
- Alcohol (at least for the first 28 days of your new dietary regime).
- All sugar-loaded fizzy drinks (soda), and all types of 'energy' drinks, often masquerading as sports beverages (switch instead to coconut water which contains high amounts of potassium, or water fortified with electrolytes).
- Restrict intake of caffeine and caffeine-based products, such as coffee and black tea (if anxiety is not an issue, caffeine in moderation can be beneficial for those with ADHD, as it can help focus attention and improve memory).
- All coffee-based drinks such as those with a bunch of artificial flavourings, colourings, sugar and whipped cream.

Chapter Takeaway

- **Medication has its place, but is often turned to first when there are other options to consider. Medical practitioners receive little if any nutritional training and so cannot be relied on for dietary advice in relation to mental health or ADHD.**

- **Nutrients are already used as aids to support mental health, such as vitamin D and omega-3 for depression.**
- **What we consume plays a big role in our moods and behaviours.**
- **ADHD symptoms are visible even in children who do not have ADHD when they consume artificial food colourings and additives.**

TAKE A STEP

Consider getting your child's nutrient levels screened with a registered nutritionist or dietician. Alternatively, start eliminating some items from the 'What to avoid' list, adding in those from the 'What to include' list.

Chapter 4

ADHD Genetics and Nutrition as a Modulator

Nutrition is something we can control, if we have the time, the information and the willpower required! But genetics also plays a role in ADHD. While you might think genetic predispositions were impossible to alter, in this chapter I discuss that even genes have some room for manipulation. Nutrition is one biological mechanism through which we may be able to turn certain aspects of genes on and off. This means that not only do food choices impact children on the gut–brain axis, but also at a cellular level, even post-birth.

I recall the British comedian Rory Bremner, who had just been diagnosed with adult ADHD at the time, asking my mentor Eric Taylor, Emeritus Professor at King's College London, during an interview if ADHD ran in families. Bremner had recognized the genetic thread in his own family and explained that his nephew's diagnosis of ADHD had been the catalyst in his own assessment. Professor Taylor explained it like this: there is not one gene but quite a number of genes, each one with a small effect contributing to different parts of the spectrum. Overall it is thought that about 80 per cent of the differences in hyperactive people come from the way genes work. Genes do not work in isolation, and the environment and genes are always at work together.

Professor Taylor then went on to describe the notion of individual variability in ADHD and how while one person will make their ADHD work for them in an intuitive and effective way, another person with ADHD may completely go under and feel they are a total failure and have a miserable time. The difference, he advised, between these two opposite scenarios depends on how other people support and help them. This, for me, was a classic example of how genes and the environment work together, and provides a simplistic example of the definition of 'epigenetics'.

There is considerable scientific evidence that nutrition is an important epigenetic factor, alongside the support system, in how someone's disposition towards ADHD traits manifests and affects them in life. Nutrition is a biological mechanism that can influence almost all of our genes; this is a field known as nutrigenomics.

Parents and professionals alike are often told that ADHD is largely 'genetic', but understanding exactly what that means is not always straightforward. In this chapter, I delve a little deeper into the meaning of a genetic condition such as ADHD, and explore the impact that environment – in the broadest sense of the word – can have on our genes. In fact, nutrition, unlike stress and other behaviours, is one of the most easily studied, and therefore better understood, environmental factors.

Everyone inherits genes from their parents, grandparents and other ancestors. These determine features such as hair and eye colour, height and susceptibility to diseases. Genes are basically types of chemicals called DNA (deoxyribonucleic acid) that are hidden inside practically every cell in our human body. They can be understood as a type of blueprint or instruction manual for who we may become. It is estimated that the human body contains around 19,000 genes – which is far less than originally thought. DNA is the carrier of genetic information, which is passed down from generation to generation.

In the last decade, we have seen advancements in genetic investigations and evidence for a brain maturation delay theory of ADHD (Rubia 2007; Shaw 2013). Other advances have been made in the field of genetics and as an outcome of large studies, such as genome-wide association studies (GWAS), that suggest an association of specific genes in the make-up of ADHD. These studies provide evidence that ADHD is highly heritable within families, with a three to five times greater risk in first-degree relations (i.e. parents, children, brothers and sisters). We now know that if a parent has ADHD, their child has a 50 per cent chance of also having it. Conversely, if your child has a diagnosis of ADHD, there is a chance that you or your partner will have it as well. In many cases genetic inheritance is responsible for ADHD's key symptoms, accounting for 70 per cent of associated hyperactive traits and 56 per cent of inattention (Nikolas and Burt 2010). A larger study based on twins put ADHD heritability levels at 76 per cent (Faraone *et al.* 2005). This still leaves a proportion of the condition unaccounted for, which can be explained by environmental factors.

The key point here, however, is that even though genetic influences are pretty sizeable, the chemical pathways involved are not yet fully mapped out or understood, and much more research is needed to better understand gene–environmental interventions.

Carly Jordan, Mum to Jordan who has ADHD, and a Blogger

There was a time, not so long ago, when medical professionals and family members didn't understand the strange behaviour and mental pain of a new mother suffering from what we now know as postnatal depression. Due to the lack of medical knowledge and a society that didn't have any other way to comprehend it, those women were sometimes horrifically locked away, silenced by prescriptive drugs, or received shocking forms of treatment and, of course, would be diagnosed as 'insane'.

Thankfully nowadays, through medical advances, we understand the hormonal changes in the body after childbirth that affect a high percentage of mothers, causing depression and, in some cases, very dangerous behaviour. Most of us understand it isn't anyone's choice to be diagnosed with a mental illness; it's out of our control and not something we can voluntarily switch on and off. We need to educate the world to understand how to support each other; we are all scared of the things we don't understand, but we can do something to change that.

ADHD is a brain-based biological disorder; it isn't a condition you 'snap out of' when you feel like it – it is a mental health disorder. Yet, despite all the science-based evidence and expert information available, we are still treating it with judgmental goggles of pure ignorance. Unfortunately, the education system and medical professionals in the UK are years behind the US in terms of specialist schools, education, treatments and support systems, mainly due to lack of funding.

Over the past seven years, I've had to attend a myriad

of frustrating meetings with teachers and medical professionals who had such archaic views on ADHD that my son was originally misdiagnosed, and this was a contributing factor in the breakdown of my marriage. Two kids and one divorce later, emotionally exhausted and fed up of listening to family members tell me things like 'He's fine, he's just a boy's boy', 'You need to set boundaries', 'He needs to pull his act together and focus' – cue the sighs of despair – I had to do something. Surely I knew my son better than anyone and needed to listen to my own intuition?

I began to research every piece of information in the US, from magazine articles, expert books written by professionals, to attending conferences and listening to any webinar I could find. Not surprisingly, everything I was learning reassured me and confirmed what I already knew – my son has ADD and anxiety. This wasn't a 'parenting' or 'laziness' issue, as most teachers would have you believe, but was down to the fact that he has an inherent neurological difference – that is, the way his brain is wired. You wouldn't say to a child in a wheelchair 'Get up and walk, and stop being lazy', and therefore, just because you can't see the disability or 'difference', don't judge or isolate someone who needs your empathy and support. We need to educate everyone, from family members to teachers, to stop hating what they don't understand.

The pain of shame is one of the most debilitating conditions associated with ADHD. This begins early on in childhood from years of negativity drummed into you from people who, through no fault of their own, just don't understand the way you are. Reaching adulthood you become defined by 'shame', low self-esteem, failing relationships, never feeling good enough, always worrying about making mistakes, leading all too often to depression. My journey with my son has led me to understand why I am the way

I am. In fact, I was misdiagnosed with depression, but I actually have ADD.

It was the light bulb moment when I realized why I struggled so much over the years, why I dropped out of so many courses, why I never finished things, why I had to be loved and be in a relationship, why I got bored so easily, why I struggled with friends, why I recently lost my job and why I hyperfocused on all the 'fun' things but never on the important things in life that we all need to focus on from time to time. There were mixed emotions of relief and guilt, and finally an understanding of why I am the way I am, and most likely why my son is the way he is. But then I realized, I am PROUD of who I am. Yes, I can be impulsive, but I am also a lot of fun. I am PROUD of my creativity even though I might be a little messy; I am PROUD of my empathy and intuition; I am PROUD to be emotional and loving; I am PROUD to be ME! Without my ADD I wouldn't have had the tenacity to keep on fighting for my son and his future. He needs me more than ever, but he also needs the world to change its perceptions.

I am hopeful, as I *do* see a slight shift in society's understanding; but it is still so small. Just as it was 60 years ago for those mothers with postnatal depression, people are still afraid of what they don't understand; people only see what they want to see; society as a whole will always prefer to ignore issues, hoping they will 'go away'. This is why it is so important to change perceptions and educate the world – knowledge is power!

ADHD is a powerful gift if understood and managed properly. We need to help individuals believe in themselves and accept their differences, but rather than focus on the negatives, we must encourage children and adults with ADHD to find solutions and systems to help them get through daily life.

Self-belief, optimism and the security of having someone to talk to is essential to success. Whether that person is a family member, a favourite teacher, a CBT (cognitive behavioural therapy) counsellor or an ADHD coach, as long as you have someone who believes in you and who is willing to listen and understand, then this will truly make all the difference.

I will always be my son's ADHD 'buddy', and it has encouraged me to return to study to become an ADHD coach, and yet, I know there are so many who don't have anyone to turn to and will most likely (statistics prove this) end up on the wrong side of the track, leading to addictions and possibly crime. We can all do something to prevent this just by opening our minds and being willing to learn about the unknown. Through education, love and support we CAN change perceptions and stop this negativity surrounding ADHD and mental health.

To other parents, I would say this: don't be ashamed – be positive, focus on your strengths, find like-minded people, and just be you.

Genes and Environment

Until fairly recently, many strands of scientific enquiry worked independently, each within a unique and often isolated domain. Geneticists studied genes, psychologists studied human behaviour and biochemists studied biochemistry. Often these fields did not openly share information or engage in collaborations. Historically, conducting scientific research was an isolating experience, with the secret note-keeping of materials and methods, and researchers frequently acting as both the test subjects and experimenters.

Fortunately, the scientific community now recognizes the need to integrate multiple strands of science such as biological, genetic and neuroimaging research to better understand the complexities of neurodevelopmental differences and psychiatric disease. It is now widely accepted that many clinical symptoms overlap with other disorders and are consequently better understood as existing on a spectrum. For example, people with ADHD are more likely to also suffer with symptoms related to depression or anxiety, and many individuals will have two or three or more diagnoses. By sharing data across diverse research programmes and clinical trials, we can learn much more about human conditions and their underlying causes.

This leads me once more to the subject of genetics and its interplay with the environment. It is thought that genetics predict a sizeable contribution in terms of our intelligence (twin studies have found a heritability of IQ between 57% and 73%, and research by Robert Plomin suggests in may be higher). However, we also know that nutrition is a contributing factor and that malnutrition (in particular insufficient amounts of iron, zinc, vitamin B and protein), especially during brain development, can lead to a loss of IQ, and increase risk for antisocial behaviour, learning problems and mood instability (Grantham-McGregor 1995). Therefore, the role of the environment is critical.

In this context, the 'environment' refers to the world we are born and socialized into, but also, prior to that, the physical environment of our mother's womb – her bodily health, nutritional status and emotional state during pregnancy and even prior to conception. There are, of course, many potential stressors in our environment that can result in genetic mutations and alter the genetic blueprint. Environmental factors that have been linked to genetic mutations include pollution, trauma, toxins (e.g. from cigarette smoke or neurotoxic chemicals), infectious diseases and nutritional deficiencies. All of these can alter our DNA.

So this is how it works: genes provide the code (or instructions) for the body to make a wide variety of different proteins (and their building blocks, amino acids) that underpin every significant biological process in our bodies. Genes receive coded instructions for making essential proteins via a process called *gene expression* (also known as 'switching on' genes) or gene silencing (also known as 'switching off' genes), since the production of different proteins will be affected by different genes being switched on and off. When modifications occur in the protein-making of genes without alterations in our original DNA sequence (our genetic code), this process is called 'epigenetics'. Basically, it's the modification of gene expression, rather than the changing of the genetic code itself.

The field of epigenetics is relatively new, emerging only in the mid-1990s, and is one of the most exciting scientific discoveries of recent times. DNA may be nature's blueprint, but it can be modified by biological markers called methyl groups (minute carbon-hydrogen instruction packs), which bind to a gene and say 'ignore this bit' or 'exaggerate this part'. Histones – a family of basic proteins that associate with DNA in the nucleus of a cell – also play a role in managing how firmly the DNA is spooled around its central thread, and consequently how decipherable the information is. It is these two epigenetic controls, comprising an on–off switch and a volume adjuster, if you like, which give each cell its commands. The addition or removal of these controls alters the expression of neighbouring genes and the very essence of the cells themselves (Carey 2012), hence how someone can have the 'genetic markers' for a disease but never contract the illness.

Epigenetics provides evidence to support the notion that genes are not static or wholly deterministic, and that there is an interactive process at play. For an analogy, think of reading the unedited script of a play that is subsequently developed as a theatre production. The outline of the play is the guide (or set of instructions), but several scenes may be deleted or replaced, meaning the entire actual theatrical production is modifiable (Carey 2012). In a similar fashion, our genetic blueprint is subject to modifications. Cells may read the script containing the genetic code, but the result is a different production, with wide implications for human health (Carey 2012). Just as DNA is capable of change, so is the structure and function of the human brain via the process of neuroplasticity, which we will come to.

For decades, there was a commonly held belief in science that the adult human brain was essentially immutable, hardwired and fixed in form and function. Furthermore, by the time we reached adulthood we were pretty much stuck with what we had. For example, it was assumed that your intelligence and personality as a child pretty much determined your abilities as an adult. Fortunately, this notion was challenged and eventually refuted in the 1960s by the pioneering work of an amazing scientist called Dr Marion Diamond. Her work demonstrated that different kinds of early life experiences led to structural changes in the brain. This discovery had sizeable implications for child development and our ability to maximize our full human potential.

Modern science has taught us that the human brain is capable of change throughout life until old age via a process called neuroplasticity. Our brain has the ability to generate new synapses – the connections between neurons that encode memories and learning – enabling people to recover from traumatic brain injury, stroke and psychiatric illness. Even the simple process of acquiring new skills – such as learning a musical instrument or a new language and/or replacing old redundant habits with new ones – changes the structure of our brain. Dr Diamond's work excited the field of neuroscience and beyond and gave everyone hope. After all, who doesn't want a better brain? Of great interest to me was the fact that the first item on her list for improving the brain was diet.

Carrie Grant, Mum, Actress, Voice Coach and TV Presenter

I have four children, three from birth, one adopted, and all with a variety of needs including Autism, Asperger's, Dyspraxia and ADHD. In fact, three of the children are diagnosed with ADHD.

I first came to know about ADHD through my oldest daughter, Olive. She went through school being told she didn't concentrate enough, she found it really hard to order her thinking, her mind constantly raced and she was always sensory-seeking. At 11 she was diagnosed with Dyspraxia. With a reading age of 18, this made sense of her writing challenges. However, the ADHD still went along hidden from school, professionals and, in our ignorance, home.

It was only when my next two daughters were diagnosed with Autism and Asperger's that I really began to look at Olive through a different lens. She certainly didn't seem to have the same challenges as the younger girls; however, as she went through her teens I began to notice there were very real differences. Her concentration was minimal unless she was doing something she was deeply interested in, and then it was off the scale. She was impulsive, would forget things, lose everything, drop everything. She would get lost, take the wrong bus or train. She was super-clever but would miss handing in assignments or miss appointments. Most of these things could be given strategies, but the hardest part was the anxiety. I became aware that she was carrying huge amounts of anxiety and this was really impacting her life. She was finally diagnosed with ADHD at the age of 18.

As parents and creatives we have encouraged her to be her unique self. We have praised her super-concentration – it's

> an advantage in many ways. We have marvelled at her brain racing – it produces creativity at an amazing rate. We have found humour in her scatteredness, and spent vast amounts of money replacing glassware. The area we have really tried to focus on is helping her to lower her anxiety. Now I look at her as an adult, self-managing, pushing through, strategied up and owning who and how she is, and I can honestly say I could not be more proud of her.

The human brain is designed to learn and the capability for learning is infinite. Let's take the notion that intelligence (IQ) is changeable. This is arguably most evident in children. Their brains are often described as being like sponges, rapidly soaking up new information via the senses from birth and beyond.

There are many studies reporting the positive effects of breastfeeding and child development. Some of these have also explored associations between breastfeeding and later intelligence (IQ), with positive findings (Ballard and Morrow 2013; Caspi *et al.* 2007; Isaacs *et al.* 2010; von Stumm and Plomin 2015). However, one large study involving 11,000 breastfed babies showed no reliable association between higher IQ and breastfeeding at age two (Chandler *et al.* 2013). So, although we may concur that breastfeeding is always best, arguably it does not conclusively predict intelligence as previously thought – the jury is still out. Of course, the nutritional composition of breast milk and the background diet of the mother should also be considered as important factors. Not all breast milk is the same, and although the general composition of water, protein, fat and lactose is common to all mothers' milk, there is individual variation, with new components still being identified (Ballard and Morrow 2013).

One large research study by scientists at the NIH in collaboration with the University of Bristol in the UK reported that eating omega-3-rich fish and seafood during pregnancy plays an important role in later child developmental outcomes, including intelligence. This data was part of the Avon Longitudinal Study of Parents and Children, which recruited over 14,000 women during pregnancy and has charted the health and development of the children ever since. The results reported that maternal seafood intake during pregnancy of less than 340g per week was associated with an increased risk of children being in the lowest quartile for verbal IQ. Additionally, children falling into the category of low or no maternal fish consumption during pregnancy were associated with increased risks of poor developmental outcomes across a wide range of measures including prosocial behaviour, fine motor, communication and social development scores (Hibbeln *et al.* 2007). This study highlighted the importance of an intake of omega-3 fatty acids during pregnancy and its potential impact on the later cognitive and social outcomes of children from age six months to eight years.

There is no doubt that nutrition plays a role here and influences the capacity to learn. For example, it can ensure the cellular structure of the brain is optimally functioning, switching on attention and optimizing mood and behaviour. The omega-3 DHA influences cell signalling across brain networks, resulting in faster and more efficient communication. Other types of omega-3 fats such as EPA (eicosapentaenoic acid) have been found to be clinically effective in reducing attention deficits and improving mood (Bloch and Qawasmi 2011; Hallahan *et al.* 2016). Nutrition, therefore, is a vehicle of change, tweaking and modifying.

Three examples follow of the interplay between genes and environment. The first example, known as the Dutch Hunger Winter, summarizes the outcome of malnutrition in a Dutch population. It has generated much interest from psychologists across the world as it highlights early epigenetic effects in a naturalistic environment (Carey 2012). A harsh winter occurred in Western Netherlands, beginning in early November 1944 and lasting until late spring in 1945. Historical records reported a bitter and cold period of famine following four years of atrocious war. The people remained under

German control and a blockade resulted in a disastrous reduction in the availability of food. This led to people trying to survive on only 30 per cent of their conventional calorie intake. More than 20,000 people died before food supplies finally reached them (Carey 2012). The effects of this period of severe malnutrition, rather unexpectedly, were far-reaching and extended beyond the immediate physical and psychological effects of the survivors.

The children of the mothers who had been pregnant during the Dutch Hunger Winter were examined, and the results were varied and unpredicted. Those babies whose mothers were malnourished only for the last few months of pregnancy were born with low birth weights and remained small for the duration of their adult lives. They also had lower rates of obesity compared to the general population. This was in spite of having access to as much food as they desired. For some reason, their bodies were unable to recover from their early exposure to malnutrition. On the other hand, the children whose mothers had been malnourished early on in pregnancy but received adequate nutrition thereafter and appeared healthy at birth went on to have elevated incidents of obesity and a greater occurrence of physical and mental health problems that affected them for decades afterwards. In some cases, the effects persisted in these children's children, as far as the great-grandchildren of the Dutch famine survivors, confirming that epigenetic effects can impact subsequent generations (Carey 2012).

A second rich data set supporting epigenetic effects comes from identical twins studies. Twins who share the same genetic code and grow in the same womb are ordinarily raised in the same home. However, studies of psychiatric illness in twins have reported that in 50 per cent of cases where one identical twin develops a serious mental illness such as schizophrenia, the other does not. Why? It's almost like a flip of a coin – heads, one escapes the disease; tails, the other suffers. Given they are identical twins, one would have thought that the genetic heritability would have been equal, but it is not (Carey 2012).

The final example I would like to share involves adoption. Imagine this common situation: a small child under three years of age who, after being exposed to neglect and abuse by his or her biological parents, is legally removed from the family home by the state and placed with loving foster or adoptive parents. The child now begins to thrive under the loving care, attention, security and stability provided in his or her new home environment. During childhood, adolescence and early adulthood, the young person stays with his or her parents. There are two possible outcomes. First, the young person experiences mental health problems, increased risk of substance abuse, self-harm, depression or anxiety and suicide attempts. Second, the young person transforms into a happy, stable individual indistinguishable from their unaffected and not adopted peers. Although the latter is possible, statistics have sadly demonstrated that the odds are unfavourably stacked against the former outcome. Even in the absence of tangible recollection of the traumatic events, early exposure to childhood trauma can have long-lasting and devastating consequences for later mental health (Carey 2012). But, we must consider that there are always 'outliers', as the author Malcolm Gladwell (2009) superbly captures in his book *Outliers: The Story of Success*.

These three examples relate to nutrition, psychiatric disease and early life trauma. They differ in theme but share one common thread – they are all examples of epigenetic effects in play. Alterations in environment can have biological consequences that persist long after the event has become a distant memory. This is the novel discipline that is revolutionizing biology and has since falsified the premature assumption that our genetic code is fully accountable for all of human life (Carey 2012). Even Charles Darwin recognized ahead of his time that there were other conditions beyond genetic inheritance and natural selection that were playing out a role:

> For natural selection acts by either now adapting the varying parts of each being to its organic and inorganic conditions of life; or by having adapted them during long-past periods of time: the adaptations being

> aided in some cases by use and disuse, being slightly affected by the direct action of the external conditions of life, and being in all cases subjected to the several laws of growth. Hence, in fact, *the law of the Conditions of Existence is the higher law*; as it includes, through the inheritance of former adaptations, that of Unity of Type. (Darwin 1859)

Environmental factors such as a habitual intake of processed and unhealthy foods, tobacco smoking, excessive alcohol consumption, psychological stress, environmental pollutants and a sedentary lifestyle can all interfere with DNA's on–off switch and contribute towards abnormal cell growth. These changes can lead to an increased risk of premature conditions such as cancer or respiratory and cardiovascular disease.[1] In a similar fashion, these alterations can affect mental health, and several molecular and biological characteristics of psychiatric diseases are consistent with epigenetic dysregulation.

Of all the modifiable environmental risk factors, the most relevant for this book is nutrition. Epigenetic research has provided evidence that specific foods, including polyunsaturated fatty acids, folate, vitamin B12, polyphenols, selenium, and certain fruits and vegetables containing natural antioxidants, have protective, inhibitory and reversible effects. There is now little doubt that certain foods have the ability to switch genes on and off. The field of epigenetics has demonstrated that nutrition is able to modify the expression of critical genes at the transcriptional level, and inhibit the development of pathologic disease processes. Many psychiatric diseases are considered to be epigenetic manifestations, and we are only just waking up to the role of adequate and healthy nutrition as a modifiable feature in the potential prevention of mental health conditions and neurodevelopmental differences (Stevens, Rucklidge and Kennedy 2017). This places humans in an empowered position as agents of their own change based on their decisions, actions and lifestyle choices.

---

1 www.who.int/nutrition/topics/4_dietnutrition_prevention/en/index4.html

The French philosopher Jean-Paul Sartre firmly adhered to the belief 'Man is nothing else but what he makes of himself.' The fact remains that the blueprint of our lives is modifiable; our DNA code can be potentially altered, and nutrition is a key modifier. To some extent this gives rise to hope and liberation from predicted scripts depending on our mind state, choices, reasoning and intellect.
In the coming chapters, you will read case studies that reflect the ability of nutrition to overcome genetics. We can act as agents of change by taking charge of the food we put into our body.

Chapter Takeaway

- **Genes and environment are always working together.**
- **Environment can alter genes by turning certain ones on and others off.**
- **Specific nutrients are brain-selective and act as agents of change, meaning that nutrition is one of the environmental factors that has the ability to modify genetics.**
- **Nutrition is the easiest environmental factor to take control of.**

TAKE A STEP

Check out your family history for signs of ADHD inheritance, and don't forget to look at yourself for possible symptoms. If you know of a relative who has ADHD or is the parent of a child with ADHD, begin a dialogue with them about the ways you've each found to manage symptoms. Perhaps prepare a recipe from the end of this book and have dinner together. If you are interested in finding out more about your DNA you can purchase a home testing kit such as the ones commercially available online: www.lifecodegx.com

Chapter 5

The Right Fat

Omega-3 Fatty Acids

In this chapter I will explain the right way to eat omega-3 fatty acids and why this is important, by explaining the significance of the conversion of short-chain polyunsaturated fatty acids (SC-PUFAs) into long-chain highly unsaturated fatty acids (LC-HUFAs). This knowledge is especially crucial for those who choose a vegan diet, as fish is the easiest source of omega-3. It's actually quite straightforward to understand, and the requisite changes in your diet or a child's diet can have an enormous impact.

Everyone always asks me: 'What worked for you, and what didn't?' Both are important questions. Just before my son was diagnosed, I was having one of those tearing-my-hair-out moments and was interrupted by a phone call from my adopted brother's old university roommate, a lovely young lady called Fatima. She had heard second-hand a little of our situation and wanted to help. It's funny how sometimes in life the *right* people enter at a time you need them most. Fatima proceeded to educate me on the role of omega-3 fish oils in ADHD.

She told me about a clinical trial that had been conducted by a scientist called Dr Alex Richardson. Funnily enough, I had heard of this researcher's name because it had been mentioned to me by my son's (very caring) SEN teacher, Eileen Howard. At that time, Fatima was working for a nutraceutical company, and asked if we would like to try some of their omega-3 fish oils. Of course I agreed. At that stage I was willing to try anything!

A small package arrived shortly after and we started on the daily recommended dose of six capsules a day, but disappointingly, with no noticeable effects. So when Fatima called again six weeks later to ask how we were getting on, I shared my observations – or lack of them! She paused and then asked, 'How much fish does your son eat?' I replied probably one portion a week – as far as fish went, he liked salmon, but not much else. Fatima said there was a possibility that he might need a higher dose, mentioning some research in the US that suggested some children with ADHD had lower blood levels of omega-3. 'Try increasing the dose to around 1 gram per day,' she advised, and so we did. To my surprise, around 10 weeks later, my son was noticeably less hyperactive and seemed calmer, to the point that other people also noticed and he said he felt 'happier'.

Every parent remembers the excitement they felt knowing they were going to have a baby. The transformation of an embryo into a foetus and then a baby is magical, and it all begins with the single rhythm of a heartbeat. This tiny little aquatic mammal then transforms into human form as it draws nourishment and energy from its mother via the placenta.

Most mothers understand that the quality of their diet is important during pregnancy. However, the unhelpful myth that pregnancy is a valid excuse to follow your cravings and eat whatever you want remains. The fact is, nutrition plays a fundamental role in determining the health of the unborn child from the word go – before conception, during the earliest stages of pregnancy, and beyond. Eating omega-3-rich foods such as fish and seafood during pregnancy has been shown to be protective against the development of ADHD-related behaviour symptoms (Sagiv *et al.* 2012).

There are certain types of foods, including omega-3 HUFAs, which can positively influence the brain, retinal function and central nervous system at various stages of the baby's development. I've mentioned one of the two key HUFAs already – DHA. The other is EPA. These can be found in various oily fish and seafood, including wild-caught salmon, fresh tuna (not canned), mackerel, herring, anchovies, sardines, shrimp, crab, lobster, oysters, mussels, clams, fish roe and cod liver oil. Supplementation is a great way of topping up, but always choose a high-quality omega-3 brand containing EPA and DHA. The dose really depends on how much fish and seafood you are already eating per week, what your omega-3 index test score is, and whether or not you have a diagnosed condition such as ADHD or depression.

Alpha-linolenic acid (also known as ALA) is a polyunsaturated fatty acid (PUFA). PUFAs are the head of the omega-3 family and ALA is plant-based. ALA is not considered a sufficient substitute for the DHA form, because it is not easily converted into the HUFAs EPA and DHA that the brain requires. ALA is, however, readily available in cooking oils such as flaxseed and rapeseed (canola) oil, and certain nuts, seeds and green leafy vegetables.

The Power of Omega-3s

Decades of evidence have confirmed that omega-3s (HUFAs) are bioactive compounds essential for neurodevelopment, brain function and structure. They are critical components of the brain's neuronal membranes and essential for a complex range of functions related to gene expression (which we learned about in the previous chapter), the production of protective sheaths around nerve fibres in the brain, communication between brain cells, and the production of dopamine (a 'pleasure' chemical). Around 25–30 per cent of all neuronal membranes are made up of these specialized and complex fats. And we're talking about a LOT of membranes – the brain contains in the region of a hundred billion neurons!

A single neuron is composed of a cell body (which contains a nucleus), dendrites (the spindly branches resembling tree-like structures that receive signals at the synapses), an axon (a medium for sending electrical messengers extending from the cell body to the end of the axon terminal) and axon terminals. Each axon is covered in a fatty sheath called myelin. This acts as an electrical insulator for the neuron and is made of the omega-3 fatty acid DHA. As mentioned in Chapter 1, DHA helps speed up cell signalling, resulting in greater brain power. Without DHA, the communication across our brains would be less efficient and slower. Omega-3s are healthy fats that are also anti-inflammatory, protecting the brain from becoming inflamed and unhealthy.

The early stages of neurodevelopment involve a number of complex processes, occurring simultaneously. Foremost amongst these are:

- Neuronal migration, the process by which neurons travel to their predestined position in the developing brain to form the cortex.
- Neurogenesis, the growth and development of neurons.
- Synaptogenesis, the formation of synapses, the connections between nerve cells.
- Myelination, the process of forming a myelin sheath around a neuron to optimize cell signalling.

All of these rely on a supply of omega-3 HUFAs.

There is now a wealth of evidence confirming the brain's requirement for increased cortical DHA concentrations during pregnancy, coinciding with very active periods of brain development in the unborn child. This maternal-to-infant LC-PUFA transport during pregnancy and lactation is a process called biomagnification (Kuipers *et al.* 2011). The richest store of LC-PUFAs is the mother's brain, and during the last trimester of pregnancy her supply is compromised in favour of her child's developing brain. This is why it is such a vital component of a mother's diet. In fact, omega-3 DHA is commonly referred to as the *building blocks* of the baby's brain and retinal function.

Most mothers can relate to the concept of experiencing 'baby brain' during the last trimester. This is thought to be directly linked to the depletion of LC-PUFAs, and is a time when the mother may become disoriented, forgetful and disorganized. She may also be feeling overly emotional and tearful. As these omega-3 fats also help regulate the neurotransmitter dopamine, which governs wellbeing and mood, the mother is at risk of the development of postnatal depression, which may begin during the last trimester.

In fact, research has shown that higher concentrations of omega-3 DHA in mothers' milk and greater seafood consumption significantly predicted lower incidences of postpartum depression (Hibbeln 2002). Another study examined the relationship between high levels of depressive symptoms in pregnancy and low omega-3 fatty acid intake from fish (Golding *et al.* 2009). The results supported an association between low omega-3 intake from seafood and an increased risk of greater depressive symptoms during pregnancy, concluding that eating seafood during pregnancy may have beneficial effects on mental wellbeing (Golding *et al.* 2009). In fact, dietary guidelines in the US were updated in 2015 to recommend that all pregnant women eat at least 340g of fish and seafood per week to preserve the neurocognitive health of their unborn child. Clinical studies have demonstrated that early dietary intervention with DHA results in improved cognitive development in infants (Dunstan *et al.* 2008; Helland *et al.* 2003; Judge, Harel and Lammi-Keefe 2007), improved visual acuity (Birch *et al.* 2002) and an improved ability in infants to problem-solve (Willatts *et al.* 1998).

Christopher Speed, MND, APD, Global Vice President of Sales and Dietitian, Wiley's Finest Wild Alaskan Fish Oil

As a dietitian and senior manager in the global supplement industry, I hold three firm beliefs about nutrition that have remained with me throughout my career and allowed me to enthusiastically work in a field that I love.

- First, inadequate dietary intake of omega-3s EPA and DHA from seafood is at the root of what makes us unwell.
- Second, our over-consumption of commoditized oils like soy has skyrocketed our omega-6 intake, leading to severe dietary essential fatty acid imbalance that further exacerbates the negative effects of omega-3 deficiency.
- Third, we can single-handedly erase most diseases of the cardiovascular system and brain by focusing on achieving optimal omega-3 intake from seafood.

These beliefs might be seen by some as improbable, but it's important to remember that omega-3s EPA and DHA are the most researched nutrients in history and we can say a more about what they do to support our wellness and health than ever before.

The profound effect omega-3s EPA and DHA have on our body and their weighty health credentials is something that has empowered the professional path I have taken. As a result, I have doggedly and determinedly tried to help people bridge one of the most pervasive nutritional inadequacies – insufficient EPA and DHA intake from seafood. Regardless of whether I have worked in clinical hospital-based environments or the commercial side of the supplement industry, I see my role to be first and foremost a scholar of nutrition where I am able to educate people on the nuances of dietary choice and how to best use food and supplements as preventive medicine. I have always felt that this is the most important thing for me to accomplish professionally, because, after all, it's the right thing to do.

For too long nutrition and preventive medicine have been shelved in the face of the current 'status quo' of modern healthcare. We need to aggressively overhaul the nutritional guidance we give the general public and make it clear that our poor diets are to blame for not just cardiovascular disease, but also mental health. Occurrences of mental ill health and brain disorders are rising in a disturbing manner and incidences of brain disorders have now overtaken heart disease throughout most of the world. We have clear proof that our brain development from the womb to the grave is intimately associated with a number of nutritional factors, most notably the type of fatty acids we consume throughout our life. Albeit far too late, the new era of dietary advice is starting to finally catch up and speak about the importance of nutrition 'from the shoulders up'.

An increasing number of healthcare professionals who are not traditionally trained in nutritional therapy are realizing the structural and functional roles that omega-3s EPA and DHA carry out in our body. A growing number of medical experts such as psychiatrists, cardiologists, haematologists, rheumatologists and immunologists are realizing that EPA and DHA affect not just classic chronic disease, but also our behavioural development, how we learn, experience life, feel pain and fight off infection. As the nutrition arena continues to prove its rightful place in standard healthcare practices, physicians will have the greatest opportunity of fulfilling their Hippocratic Oath to treat the ill to the best of their ability underpinned by the best scientific knowledge, especially as it relates to optimal nutrition. With our current understanding of nutrition getting stronger and fields of epigenetic research growing, the old adage 'we are what we eat' couldn't be more truthful than what we experience today.

This is why I believe the omega-3 supplementation industry is so important from a public health standpoint and should be embraced by all healthcare professionals. We provide an excellent solution for most people who are simply not willing or able to achieve adequate nutrient intake via whole foods. Very few of us consume ample fatty fish each day that would provide us with the essential benefits of omega-3s EPA and DHA. Being able to plug this gap with a supplement that is safe, affordable and simple is the perfect solution for most people on the planet.

I applaud the work of individuals like Dr Rachel Gow who shine a light on health-related problems that suffer from social stigma, and respect her passion to offer plausible nutritional solutions to prevent, control or ameliorate a range of disorders. I appreciate anyone who can comprehend the complexities of neuroscience and from this determine solutions for people so that they are given the very best chance of thriving throughout their life.

Arguably, the largest body of evidence for oiling the brain with omega-3 fats originates from clinical trials in both ADHD and depression.

One of the main mechanisms of action of omega-3 fats in the brain is their role in regulating neurotransmitters responsible for our mood and wellbeing: namely serotonin, often referred to as 'the happiness chemical,' and dopamine, 'the pleasure chemical'. Dopamine not only gives us feelings of immense pleasure – it also affects our movement, mental alertness and sensations of pain. The production of dopamine is reliant on a dietary intake of omega-3 fatty acids. In fact, studies have persistently shown that a lack of these omega-3 HUFAs reduces the amount of dopamine available in the brain. Dopamine plays a critical role in the way our brain responds to reward and is produced after most pleasurable acts, such as eating a favourite meal or winning a race or a game.

Alterations in dopamine or a reduction in dopamine levels will affect the way we respond to rewards and other pleasurable acts, and low levels can result in unhappiness, leading to depression, a lack of motivation, forgetfulness, irritability, mood swings and a lack of concentration. In addition, you may develop ADHD-type symptoms and suffer with fatigue. Low intake of essential omega-3 HUFAs can significantly deplete dopamine in the brain and alterations in dopamine neurotransmission (Bondi *et al.* 2013; Chalon 2006). Researchers working in the field of nutritional psychiatry recognize that eating fish and seafood at least twice a week will help ensure an adequate intake of omega-3 and therefore optimize the neurotransmitter function and the regulation of dopamine.

Professor Robert McNamara conducted the first brain-imaging dietary intervention study in 2010. This clinical trial used fMRI to examine the brain activity of 38 healthy boys aged eight to ten while they were doing a task that measured their ability to maintain attention. The children were randomly allocated to receive omega-3 DHA in two differing dose groups – 12 of the children received 400mg per day, 14 received 1200mg, and 12 were given a placebo. The boys had two fMRI scans at the start of the trial prior to supplementation and then at the end of the trial at eight weeks.

Both groups of children taking DHA showed increased activation of the region of the brain linked to attention processes. As blood levels of DHA increased, brain activation also increased. The findings also reported that as levels of omega-3 DHA *increased*, the children's reaction time *decreased*. In other words, they became faster and performance was improved.

Additionally, a growing body of research has suggested a role for omega-3 fats as an alternative or additional treatment for ADHD, with evidence coming from four main sources:

- The animal literature, demonstrating clear effects of omega-3 deficiencies in the brain (Chalon 2006; Levant, Radel and Carlson 2004; Zimmer *et al.* 2000).
- Published research examining omega-3 blood compositions in children and young adults with ADHD and comparing it to age- and sex-matched controls (Hawkey and Nigg 2014). The collective evidence has persistently reported lower levels of omega-3 in children and young adults with ADHD, and in some instances, elevated levels of omega-6 (more on this fatty acid in the next section).
- Epidemiological evidence from several countries (epidemiology is the branch of science that contends with the incidence, distribution and control of disease in a population) examining dietary/nutrient patterns and the prevalence of ADHD. The findings are that symptoms and/or diagnoses are generally lower for Mediterranean-type or 'traditional' dietary patterns (that is, those richer in omega-3, and sometimes also omega-6), and higher for diets rich in highly processed, sugary and/or 'fast food' (Ríos-Hernández *et al.* 2017; Zhou *et al.* 2016). Furthermore, the modern Western diet or SAD (Standard American Diet) is also linked to poorer cognitive performance in school children aged six to eight (Haapala *et al.* 2015) and structural alterations in the adult brain, namely, a smaller hippocampus (the part of the brain critical for memory, learning and the generation of new cells) (Jacka, Cherbuin and Butterworth 2015).
- Meta-analytic reviews, which pool data from clinical trials into a large data set and reanalyse the data to establish an overall effect size. Several studies have now reported beneficial effects of omega-3 supplements in reducing clinical symptoms of ADHD (e.g. inattention, restlessness,

disorganization, concentration, hyperactivity and impulsivity), with EPA-rich formulations appearing to have greater efficacy (Bloch and Hannestad 2012; Hawkey and Nigg 2014; Puri and Martins 2014; Sonuga-Barke *et al.* 2013).

The Omega-3/Omega-6 Imbalance

Omega-6 is a different compound to omega-3; in fact, it competes with omega-3 in order to acquire space in the cells of our body and brain. The average person following a Western-type diet is estimated to be consuming between 12 and 17 grams of omega-6 daily. This means that the ratio of omega-3 and omega-6 in the brain will be unbalanced, with the latter taking more of the space (Simopoulos 2016).

As omega-6 fats are pro-inflammatory, an excess of them in modern Western diets has serious implications. The concern is not only for brain health, but also for various physical health conditions, premature disease and the development of obesity and type 2 diabetes (Simopoulos 2002). This is not to dispute the importance of omega-6 for the brain – all cells require it – but it is the *balance* that is critical. Scientists have estimated that the correct balance of omega-6 to omega-3 is 2:1 or 1:1 (the optimal balance for brain health). Current estimates suggest that this ratio in most Americans is more in the region of 20:1 (Simopoulos 2016).

This alarming imbalance is due to an excessive consumption of omega-6-rich foods, predominately via the inclusion of soybean oil in practically all commercially produced, processed supermarket foods. Westernized diets, including SAD, are now overloaded in omega-6 linoleic acid (LA), leading to a biochemical imbalance in our brains, which, in turn, can lead to chronic inflammation with serious consequences for mental health.

Researchers at the NIH published a paper in 2011 highlighting the dramatic rise and over-representation of omega-6 LA in our diet, mainly via the consumption of soybean oil, the results revealing a staggering 1163-fold increase between 1909 and 1999 (Blasbalg *et al.* 2011). This influx of LA-rich, cheap industrially refined and hydrogenated oils and cheap bulk processed foods are hypothesized by many scientists, including Barry Sears (author of *Toxic Fat*, 2008) and David Perlmutter (author of *Grain Brain*, 2013), to have led to inflammation in the brain (see Perlmutter and Loberg 2013; Sears 2008) and the premature development of metabolic disease. This biochemical imbalance of omega-3 and omega-6 in the brain is theorized to have contributed to the worldwide pandemic we now face of premature type 2 diabetes, Alzheimer's, obesity, brain disorders including poor mental health, and much, much more. Diets low in omega-3 fats and high in omega-6 fats are linked to higher levels of neurodevelopmental deficits, violent crime, homicide and suicide (Gow and Hibbeln 2014; Hibbeln 2007; Hibbeln and Gow 2014). The US Centers of Disease Control and Prevention have reported that 18.8 Americans were diagnosed with diabetes in 2010, with an additional 7 million cases going undetected. Between 1995 and 2010, the number of diagnosed patients increased by 50 per cent or more across 42 states, and by 100 per cent or more in 18 states.

To sit back and pretend this is not related to diet is a fundamental mistake.

Soybean oil is one of the most abundantly used vegetables oils in the Western world (the others are palm, rapeseed (canola) and sunflower). Even animals such as chickens and hens reared in industrial factory farms are fed soybean oil pellets. The main ingredient in soybean is the omega-6 LA, which is head of the omega-6 family of PUFAs. Through various biochemical processes, an excessive intake of omega-6 can increase risk of brain inflammation, which, in turn, is thought to contribute to the development of depression and other psychiatric diseases.

The important message here is that there is little point taking a 1g fish oil capsule per day and thinking that this will suffice. In fact, it probably won't even make a dent if you are eating a traditional Western diet (junk food and processed foods including cheap vegetable oils and cheap refined carbohydrates) because that 1g fish oil capsule of EPA or DHA will likely be competing against a very large backdrop of omega-6 LA. The answer is to substantially decrease your intake of omega-6-rich foods while at the same time increasing your intake of omega-3-rich foods.

For example, feeding our children cod fish fingers (fish sticks) is *not* going to provide any omega-3, unless they have been enriched with it. In addition, the breadcrumbs the fish is coated in are likely to contain rapeseed (canola) oil, which is made of omega-6. You can replace those cod fish fingers with an omega-3-enriched variety, or better still, make your own delicious fish goujons using strips of boneless fresh salmon, tuna or halibut. Most children won't even notice the difference!

The Seafood Battle

The main way to increase your intake of omega-3 is by eating fish and in particular, oily fish. There's no easy way around this, and if you have a 'fussy eater' to contend with, along with an ADHD-related behaviour management issue, it may seem as if there is a mountain ahead. But, like most mountains, it can easily turn out to be a molehill, with a dose of strategy and planning. As I recommended before, try replacing the fish fingers (fish sticks) with your own homemade omega-3-enriched version. Try using fresh tuna (cooked) in place of the tinned variety when you make tuna mayonnaise (or use cooked fresh wild salmon instead). Prepare fish cakes using a mixture of different fish, including an oily one such as mackerel. Sneak some crab meat or finely chopped prawns into your pasta sauce. Anchovies are fantastic in sauces too, enhancing flavour rather than taking over. Replace the traditional beef taco with a fish taco – taco flavours are quite strong and can easily obscure the fishiness. Above all, lead by example and normalize the eating of fish and seafood as early as possible.

Which brings me to a key point. Please pause and ask yourself, how many portions of oily fish and seafood do *you* currently eat, and how often? When parents visit my clinic to have their child's omega-3 levels tested, I often suggest they check out their levels too. Often parents will have lower omega-3 indexes than their child, placing them in an *at risk* category for poor cardiovascular and brain health. It is recommended that we eat at least two pieces of oily fish per week to receive adequate amounts of essential omega-3 fats. And it's not just about omega-3 fats either. A piece of fish also contains other vital nutrients such as zinc, magnesium, iron, iodine, selenium, copper, potassium, vitamins B6 and B12 and vitamin D – some of which will help the absorption of omega-3 into your cells.

Encouraging children to eat oily fish may take time, especially if you introduce it later in childhood. However, it is absolutely critical, and there are many recipes for seafood and fish meals at the end of this book. I recommend conducting an omega-3 finger-prick test to assess your blood levels. This will check your red blood cell EPA and DHA percentage composition and provide you with an index score ranging from 0–4 per cent as suboptimal, 4–8 per cent as intermediate and 8–12 per cent as ideal. (Tests are commercially available and can be conducted simply at home.)

James R. Dick, Nutrition Analytical Service, Institute of Aquaculture, University of Stirling, Scotland

The potential health benefits of consuming n-3 LC-PUFAs are now well recognized and there is a significant body of literature describing the health benefits of increasing our intake of LC-n-3 PUFAs, especially with respect to inflammatory pathologies, particularly for cardiovascular disease, immune function and rheumatoid arthritis (Bjørkkjær *et al.* 2006; Calder 2010; Lee *et al.* 1991; Micallef and Garg 2009).

Principally, omega-3 is derived from marine invertebrates that are consumed by fish and other marine organisms and are passed on up the aquatic food chain to a range of fish species. While all fish species contain omega-3, it is the oily fish that deposit the highest levels of it in their tissue and that can provide the highest levels of EPA and DHA to human consumers. The fish species with the highest levels of omega-3 include Atlantic and Pacific salmon, mackerel, herring and trout as well as smaller species such as sardines, anchovies and sprats. Omega-3 supplementation can also be provided from processed oil capsules.

There have also been developments regarding the impact of omega-3 supplementation in infants, especially with respect to DHA, which is vital for neural development, retinal function and nerve growth. Thus, consumption of oily fish and/or omega-3 capsules during pregnancy can improve the early development of infants as well as older children (Forsyth *et al.* 2003; Richardson and Montgomery 2005).

Reduced concentrations of both DHA and EPA have been reported in children with developmental disorders, including Autism and ADHD, but there is also evidence that supplementation with LC-n-3 PUFAs might be beneficial for children in general. Evidence from clinical trials suggests that supplementation with DHA and EPA can improve general child learning and behaviour (Richardson *et al.* 2012).

A study that links fish consumption, death rates and cardiovascular disease by the Harvard School of Public

Health (HSPH) and the University of Washington (Mozaffarian *et al.* 2013) found that older adults with higher blood levels of omega-3 fatty acids from fish and seafood had less than a 25 per cent less chance of dying prematurely than those with low omega-3 levels. Those who ate oily fish twice per week could live up to two years longer, with higher levels of omega-3 fatty acids also found to reduce the likelihood of dying from coronary heart disease by as much as 40 per cent and heart arrhythmias by 45 per cent.

Scientists at the University of Stirling's Institute of Aquaculture have collaborated with scientific companies as well as industry suppliers to provide a rapid omega-3 blood analysis report that is available to a wide range of people, including individual patients and high-performance athletes, as well as clinical studies conducted by pharmaceutical companies and related organizations.

This finger-prick blood test measures the level of omega-3 in the blood, and determines the individual requirement of this super-nutrient needed to improve one's health. The test measures the vital balance of omega-3 and omega-6 fats in the body, taking the guesswork out of omega-3 supplementation. It provides a non-invasive method of sampling blood, which can be especially important when dealing with vulnerable groups such as the young, the elderly and patients with behavioural disorders.

The ability to measure the omega-3 status of any individual at any time should prove invaluable when evaluating any health-related issue, whether in a clinical trial or as a measure of good health and wellbeing. It should be on everyone's agenda to know 'What's my score?'

Chapter Takeaway

- **Omega-3 fatty acids are brain essential for many biological functions, including dopamine production, protection of nerve fibres, gene expression and communication between brain cells.**
- **Many studies have found lower blood levels of omega-3s in children and young adults with ADHD.**
- **Omega-3s and omega-6s are both essential, but they are in competition. It's best to have a ratio of 2:1 or 1:1 (omega-6 to omega-3) for optimal brain health. Modern diets favour omega-6s and can range from a ratio of 16:1 to 20:1 (Simopoulos 2002).**
- **For brain health and as treatment for ADHD, try to up omega-3s while lowering omega-6s. The easiest way to do this is to consume oily fish and seafood at least twice a week and to decrease or eliminate those foods that contain omega-6s (found in soybean, palm, rapeseed (canola) and sunflower oil).**

TAKE A STEP

Get your own and/or your child's blood tested for omega-3 levels. As noted, these tests are commercially available and can be done at home. Additionally, start replacing foods rich in omega-6 with those that contain more omega-3. Instead of canned tuna, use fresh, or instead of cod fish fingers (fish sticks), make fish goujons using strips of boneless fresh salmon, tuna or halibut.

Chapter 6

Other Nutrients for Coping with ADHD

The growing field of nutritional psychiatry recognizes that a wide range of nutrients including vitamins A and B, choline, folate, iron, zinc, copper, iodine and omega-3s are vital for healthy brain function, wellbeing, mood and behaviour. We've already established that evidence from clinical trials has confirmed the role of omega-3 fats in improving symptoms related to ADHD, but other nutrients are also notable when it comes to improving brain health and managing ADHD.

As much as possible I encourage the families I work with to have their children's nutrient intake assessed. I work closely with a laboratory in London to facilitate this, and I have created a bespoke package for my clients based on key nutrients directly or indirectly linked to brain function. This includes testing reference intakes of the following:

- Magnesium: good sources include dark chocolate, avocado, almonds, cashews, legumes, sesame and pumpkin seeds, brown rice, chard (silver beet), broccoli, bananas, fish.
- Iodine: good sources include fish and seafood, eggs, seaweed, prunes.
- Vitamin A: good sources include organic beef and lamb liver, oily fish such as fresh salmon and tuna, cheese, eggs, tomatoes, orange and yellow vegetables.
- Vitamin C: good sources include citrus fruits, kiwifruit, strawberries, pineapples, papayas, peppers (bell peppers), broccoli, kale, tomatoes.
- Vitamin E: good sources include sunflower seeds and sunflower oil, green leafy vegetables, almonds, hazelnuts, Brazil nuts, pine nuts, peanuts, wild salmon, trout, goose, duck, avocado, mango.
- Carotene: good sources include carrots, cantaloupe, winter squash, sweet potatoes, turnips, tomatoes, spinach, kale, plums, pumpkin, apricots, egg yolks.
- Vitamin B1 (also known as thiamine): good sources include wheat germ, oats (oatmeal), beef from cows that have been grass-fed, tuna, trout, seafood, oranges, eggs, legumes, peas, nuts, seeds.
- Vitamin B2 (also known a riboflavin): good sources include quinoa, salmon, seafood, beef from cows that have been grass-fed, poultry, eggs, spinach, legumes, avocado, broccoli, nuts, seeds.
- Vitamin B6: good sources include poultry, fish, oats (oatmeal), wheat germ, brown rice, eggs, legumes, nuts.
- Vitamin B12: good sources include liver and kidney, clams, tuna, sardines, trout, beef from cows that have been grass-fed, eggs, dairy.

- Folic acid (also known as folate): good sources include legumes, peas, beans, lentils, asparagus, leafy greens, Brussels sprouts, broccoli, beetroot (beets), citrus fruit, eggs.

You might notice that, once again, fish and seafood are huge providers of many essential brain nutrients. In the test I also take an omega-3 and omega-6 fatty acids profile, and importantly, an Inge Food 'Allergy' and an IgG Food 'Intolerance' screen (more on this in the next chapter). At a minimum, I always encourage an omega-3 finger-prick test, which can be self-administered.

I would like to share with you that 100 per cent of the families I have worked with thus far whose children have been tested have presented with a wide range of nutritional insufficiencies and levels below recommended daily reference intakes – as well as food allergies/intolerances. All of these children and young adults had behavioural and/or mood disturbances, and a clinical diagnosis of ADHD, Autism or some other type of learning and behaviour difference.

I frequently share nutritional advice with the families I work with, and I even managed to get a donation of omega-3 supplements for a Brixton-based children's community centre. This charity ran a campaign called 'The Plate Pledge' that aimed at raising funds so that every child visiting would at the very least receive a hot meal. Alongside staff at head office, we designed a nutritional survey on the eating habits of the families who attended the centres. The results revealed that in this cohort of inner-city London children, 77 per cent were hungry most of the time and 64 per cent reported that there was no food at home. Meanwhile, in an anonymous survey of London schools, 78.8 per cent of head teachers and pastoral staff felt that poor nutrition was contributing negatively towards children's behaviour. A UK study conducted by Dr Charlotte Evans and researchers (2018) at the University of Leeds reported that just under 20 per cent of primary school children were not meeting the recommended intakes of iron, zinc, calcium and folic acid. The link between a child's nutritional status, learning and behaviour warrants much better attention.

Professor Margaret Rayman and Sarah C. Bath, Department of Nutritional Sciences, Faculty of Health and Medical Sciences, University of Surrey, UK

The importance of iodine adequacy in pregnancy for brain development in infants

Our research in the Department of Nutritional Sciences studies the role of specific nutrients in pregnancy, the developing brain and beyond. Iodine is critical in early brain development (Iodine Global Network 2017; Knudsen *et al.* 2000; WHO, UNICEF and ICCIDD 2007; Zimmermann 2009), and is a key constituent of the thyroid hormones. It is sourced from foods such as seaweed, fish, eggs and prunes. Pregnant women are at high risk of iodine deficiency as their intake requirements are at least 50 per cent higher than in the pre-pregnant state (WHO *et al.* 2007). This puts the developing infant at risk as the pregnant mother is its sole source of iodine for thyroid hormone production.

How is iodine status measured?

Iodine status is usually measured by urinary iodine concentration (UIC) in a spot urine sample (Iodine Global Network 2017; Knudsen *et al.* 2000; WHO *et al.* 2007; Zimmermann 2009). However, owing to variation in day-to-day iodine intake and hydration status, this measurement cannot be applied to an individual (WHO *et al.* 2007; Zimmermann 2009). Hydration status can be corrected for in adults by dividing UIC by urinary creatinine (Creat) concentration to give UI:Creat, on the basis that in a group of same sex and age, the amount of creatinine excreted per day is constant (Knudsen *et al.* 2000).

Iodine deficiency in pregnant women is common and affects child cognitive function

The 2017 Iodine Global Network map and scorecard of iodine nutrition in pregnant women shows that deficiency is common in many countries (Iodine Global Network 2017), including the UK (Bath and Rayman 2015; Iodine Global Network 2017; Knight *et al.* 2017). Our group has shown a significant negative association between mild-to-moderate iodine deficiency (measured by UIC:Creat) in first-trimester UK pregnant women from the Avon Longitudinal Study of Parents and Children cohort and children's IQ and reading ability at age eight to nine (Bath *et al.* 2013). Other studies in regions of mild-to-moderate deficiency have also found an association between poorer iodine status and adverse cognitive development, poorer working memory and poorer spelling (Abel *et al.* 2017; Costeira *et al.* 2011; Hynes *et al.* 2013).

How can women ensure that they enter pregnancy with adequate iodine status?

Food sources of iodine are somewhat dependent on location, although seafood, most notably haddock, cod, crab, large/Dublin Bay prawns (often called scampi), is generally a rich source (Bath and Rayman 2016; NIH n.d.; PHE 2015). Many countries have salt fortified with iodine, although this is not the case in the UK, where such fortified salt is difficult to find. In the UK, as in many countries, milk and dairy products are the main dietary source, with eggs also providing a useful amount of iodine (Bath and Rayman 2016; NIH n.d.; PHE 2015). Women who do not consume dairy products or seafood and who have access to iodized salt should consider a daily supplement containing 140–150µg iodine, particularly if planning pregnancy (Bath and Rayman 2016; NIH n.d.; PHE 2015). Although high in iodine, intake of brown seaweed (e.g. kelp or kombu), or brown seaweed supplements, should be avoided pre-conception as their iodine content can reach toxic levels (Yeh, Hung and Lin 2014). Advice on iodine sources can be found in the Iodine Food Fact Sheet, published by the British Dietetic Association (BDA) (Bath and Rayman 2016).

Is it sufficient to start increasing iodine intake or to supplement with iodine once pregnancy has been confirmed?

A recent UK study has shown that the children of women with pre-conception iodine deficiency, defined as UI:Creat <50µg/g, when compared with the children of iodine-adequate women, UIC:Creat ≥150µg/g, had an IQ that was lower at age six to seven by 7.5 IQ points (Robinson *et al.* 2018). This study points to the fact that women need to be iodine-adequate at a very early stage of pregnancy, indeed, before they know they are pregnant. All women of childbearing age need to be made aware of the importance of iodine.

A Case in Point

Let's look at Sarah and her son Lucas. Sarah first contacted me as her son Lucas had just been diagnosed with ADHD and she was reluctant to start him on medication as he was just six years old at the time. Her ultimate goal was to improve her son's diet, and, through those dietary improvements, help enhance his focus and attention at school.

Following a referral for nutrient testing, the results revealed Lucas had several moderate and high food allergies. In addition, Lucas presented with nutritional insufficiencies in vitamins D, B2, iodine, zinc and iron, as well as having a low omega-3 index.

This is just a single example of how drastic these invisible nutritional deficiencies can be. These results have important implications for brain function. For example, insufficient levels of zinc are linked to behavioural disturbances in motor and cognitive function as well as poor attention and lower alertness.

In several research studies, supplementation with zinc has been found to improve hyperactivity and impulsive behaviour (but not attention measures) in children with ADHD when compared to a placebo (Bilicia *et al.* 2004). One 2005 review looked at nine studies of children with ADHD and reported low zinc levels in all of them as well as a link between lower levels and the severity of symptoms (Arnold and DiSilvestro 2005). However, well-controlled zinc supplementation studies in children with ADHD are scarce, despite findings of lower blood levels in children with ADHD compared to undiagnosed control children (Dodig-Curković *et al.* 2009). Given zinc is also vital for the absorption of other nutrients, this may contribute to suboptimal levels of other nutrients intakes such as omega-3 (Huss, Völp and Stauss-Grabo 2010; Salehi *et al.* 2016).

Iron is critical for normal growth and development and for cognitive, motor and social-emotional function (Beard and Connor 2003; Georgieff 2008; Lozoff *et al.* 2006). Lower iron levels are also linked to ADHD (Grantham-McGregor and Ani 2001). Critically, iron deficiency (ID) is known to disrupt brain levels of dopamine as well as play a role in the development of restless leg syndrome (Coe *et al.* 2009). In fact, behaviours that are dependent on dopamine such as motivation, reward- and emotion-related processes are key issues in ID (Lozoff 2007). Furthermore, ID has been identified as the leading nutrition-related cause of impaired child development, while correction contributes to better child development (McCann and Ames 2007; Sachdev, Gera and Nestel 2005). Of course, we know that low omega-3 is linked to ADHD (Gow and Hibbeln 2014; Hawkey and Nigg 2014), depression (Freeman *et al.* 2006, 2010; Hallahan *et al.* 2016) and poor sleep (Montgomery *et al.* 2014; Peirano *et al.* 2009), and supplementation in several clinical trials and meta-analytic reviews has improved some of these parameters. Insufficient levels of vitamin D are linked to low mood, depression and anxiety (Spedding 2014). Research by Kamal, Berner and Ehlayel (2014) reported significantly lower vitamin D levels in 1331 children and adolescents, aged between 5 and 18, who were diagnosed with ADHD compared to healthy control children. Vitamin D deficiency was also higher in those children with ADHD compared to the non-diagnosed control children. Low concentrations of vitamin B2 (riboflavin) as well as B6 (pyridoxine) and B9 (folic acid/folate) have been found in individuals with ADHD, and lower concentrations of vitamins B2 and B6 have been associated with higher ADHD symptom scores (Landaas *et al.* 2016).

We will return to Sarah and Lucas' story in the next chapter, but for now, you can see that there were lots of ways to improve Lucas' diet, and many of them are linked to ADHD symptoms.

A Word about Supplements

The role of supplementation is quite simply to supplement your daily diet! While supplementation is never better than eating the actual nutrient-rich foods, they can help to correct insufficient levels and be useful in cases of extreme fussy eating. This is my advice: if and when you start any new nutritional programme, depending on the quality of your current diet, it is advisable to supplement in the first six to eight weeks to build up immunity and to correct any nutritional insufficiencies your child (or you yourself) may have.

But please follow RULE NUMBER 1 and find out what the child's (and your) nutrient status and numbers are! You can do this either privately under the guidance of a qualified nutritionist or dietician, or ask your family medical practitioner. You need to know where you're starting out from (in other words – your baseline level pre-intervention) before you can improve; plus you don't want to be wasting money on supplements you don't need if you're receiving sufficient amounts from your diet.

Here are a few recommendations for supplementation:

- Omega-3 fats can be taken as fish oil capsules or a smoothie emulsion, but don't just pick any brand name – choose a brand that contains both EPA and DHA.
- B1 (thiamine), especially for all those who drink alcohol, which depletes the body's store of thiamine, increasing your risk of thiamine deficiency and altering the function of the central nervous system. Symptoms of B1 insufficiency can range from fatigue, loss of appetite, irritability and poor memory to impaired cognitive performance.
- Vitamin D, especially in the winter months (November to March). Around 65 per cent of people in the UK are estimated to be vitamin D deficient, which can increase the risk of depression and anxiety. Capsules and/or an oral spray are available in all reputable health food stores.
- Greens alkaline supplements (e.g. organic chlorella and spirulina). These are natural algae containing healthy bacteria, 'cyanobacteria', which are high in protein and rich in antioxidants, B vitamins and other health-boosting nutrients including beta-carotene, iron, manganese and vitamin A.
- Vitamins and minerals containing at least some of the following: B2, B6, B12, zinc, selenium, copper, magnesium, manganese.

- Vitamin C, if you or your child is not eating at least five portions of fruit and vegetables a day. An adequate supply is necessary for the health and repair of a range of bodily tissues including teeth and gums, bone and cartilage. Vitamin C also helps maintain healthy skin and the immune system. A lack of vitamin C can cause tiredness, bleeding and deterioration of the gums, joint and muscle ache, infections, dry hair and skin, and mood changes (e.g. irritability) among other symptoms.
- Vitamin E: insufficient levels are linked to neurological and visual impairments and muscle weakness. Low levels are also associated with a weakened immune system.
- Prebiotics and probiotics: prebiotics are indigestible plant fibres residing in the intestines, and probiotics are live microorganisms (generally different strains of bacteria) to help promote healthy gut flora. Remember that gut–brain axis? It is estimated that 80 per cent of serotonin is made in the digestive tract, and healthy gut microbiota are necessary for its production. Remember, improving gut health = improving brain health.
- DIFALA is a natural alkalizing detox edible clay supplement. One of its main ingredients is clipnoptilolite, a natural zeolite (volcanic mineral) that helps remove any heavy metals and other environmental chemicals out of the system. It also contains Jamaican herbs including soursop leaves, dandelion, cow tongue flower, moringa, wheatgrass, flaxseed and spirulina.

It is always important to work with your diet first and get a good idea of your numbers (daily recommended reference intakes). However, supplementing is often needed for the first six to eight weeks, especially if there has been a lack of fruits, vegetables and omega-3 fats in the diet. If you recall, a diet high in omega-6 can basically negate any omega-3 supplement taken. Nutrients do not tend to work in isolation. They work in synergy to optimize absorption; therefore sourcing nutrients directly from food (especially seafood and oily fish) provides a greater variety of nutrients which work together.

Chapter Takeaway

- **In addition to omega-3s, several other nutrient deficiencies are linked to poor mental health; these include zinc, iron and vitamins D, B2, B6, B9 and B12.**
- **In my own work with children and young adults, I have seen the beneficial role of nutrition in child behaviour and mood, especially in those with ADHD.**
- **It's best to get nutrients from foods. However, early on in a new nutrition programme, you may require supplementation to help certain nutrient levels recover.**
- **I recommend nutrient testing before beginning any supplementation.**

TAKE A STEP

Consider having a full nutrient evaluation for your child and/or yourself, or if you are working with a family, suggest they do this. Check the list at the beginning of this chapter for nutrients you or they may need to increase, and start incorporating some of the food sources listed for those nutrients into the family's diet.

Chapter 7

Food Allergies and Sensitivities

Alongside the nutrients that can be beneficial for ADHD, it is important to be aware of food allergies and sensitivities. Children react differently to different foods, and these reactions are defined as either food *allergies* or food *intolerances*. Food allergies trigger the immune system, while food intolerance does not. Some children will experience digestive problems after eating certain foods, even though their immune system has not reacted; in other words, there is no histamine response. So allergic reactions are caused by the immune system and intolerance reactions are not.

In many cases a food intolerance is caused by the lack of an enzyme. Taking cow's milk as an example, children who are lactose intolerant will not produce enough lactase. This is an enzyme that breaks down milk sugar, called lactose, into smaller molecules that the body can further break down and absorb via the intestine. Any remaining lactose in the digestive tract can cause bloating, diarrhoea, spasms, stomach aches and gas. Those with an *allergy* to milk protein have comparable symptoms to those suffering with *lactose intolerance*, which is why lactose-intolerant individuals are commonly misdiagnosed as allergic.

Signs and symptoms of allergies and intolerances often overlap, making it difficult to distinguish between the two, although food intolerance symptoms are not always obvious and can go unnoticed for longer periods of time. Foods most commonly associated with food intolerance include casein (milk protein), cow's milk, yoghurt, cheese and other dairy products, egg yolks, egg whites, wheat, wheat gluten and other grains that contain gluten, and foods that cause intestinal gas build-up, such as beans and cabbage. Typical symptoms may include digestive issues (bloating, stomach upset, stomach-ache, gas), migraine or headache, cough, runny nose, generally feeling under the weather, and hives or rashes.

Food allergies and intolerances can also affect the central nervous system, bladder, eyes, heart, skin and musculoskeletal system. In terms of mental health they are linked to anxiety and mood disturbances including panic attacks; depression; irritability and tearfulness; oppositional behaviours such as aggression, temper tantrums and argumentative behaviour; poor coordination affecting handwriting and clumsy behaviour; memory, concentration and attention; and speech and language, including selective mutism and sleep problems (Richardson 2006).

Individuals with ASD and ADHD tend to suffer from gastrointestinal problems – reflux, vomiting, bloating, diarrhoea, abdominal pain and constipation. Their food allergy-related symptoms are not restricted to the gastrointestinal tract but can also occur in the airways and the skin – for example, behavioural problems are twice as high in children with asthma (McQuaid, Kopel and Nassau 2001). Allergic immune reactions and adverse reactions to certain food types appear frequently in children with ASD and ADHD.

Parents of children with ASD, which, as we have seen, can sometimes co-occur with ADHD, report that their children suffer from food allergies far more than non-diagnosed children (Chandler *et al.* 2013; Gurney, McPheeters and Davis 2006). Common food allergies reported include peanut, soy, wheat, gluten and dairy. Parents can be completely unaware that their child has nutritional insufficiencies and/or food intolerances, as symptoms are not always obvious and symptoms such as dry cracked skin, fatigue, anxiety, attention deficits, stomach pain or headaches are frequently dismissed. As a result, the link between behavioural and mood symptoms and the foods children are eating is far too often overlooked.

Quite often a general medical practitioner will follow a short online checklist with the patient and, based on the results, a prescription is issued then and there. However, what is strikingly apparent, and concerning, is that during these diagnostic evaluations, food allergies and intolerances, and the presence of nutritional insufficiencies of key micronutrients known to impact neurotransmitter functions, are *not* taken into consideration or assessed. A simple referral to a dietician or registered nutritionist would reveal if the presenting behaviours are truly due to ADHD or are, instead, a direct cause of food-related issues. Within my own private practice, clients seek help for nutrition-related interventions to tackle their child's symptoms of ADHD, ASD or other mood or behavioural conditions, and I always encourage them to have the child tested for food allergies and food intolerances. So far, I have not had *one* child who has not presented with some type of nutritional insufficiency and/or food intolerance or allergy.

As part of my psychological and nutritional consultation service, I created a bespoke screening package for clients, using blood samples, to test for a wide range of nutritional insufficiencies, food intolerances and allergies. The point being, in my opinion, that if you don't take a baseline assessment based on blood analysis, you are really fumbling around in the dark, and you can't possibly provide nutritional recommendations based on thin air. Blood data in my mind is the answer! It enables us to make personalized, evidence-based nutrition plans to correct insufficiencies and to avoid foods you or your child is either intolerant or allergic to.

Remember Sarah and her son Lucas? Lucas' moderate and high food intolerances included gliadin (which belongs to a class of proteins present in wheat and cereals and is a component of gluten), casein (found in dairy products), eggs (both the yolk and the white), wheat and gluten. Sarah has since worked hard to correct his nutrient insufficiencies by making changes to Lucas' diet and supplementing where necessary. She eliminated (for a period of time) foods such as gluten, wheat and dairy, which Lucas was intolerant to, and topped up his diet with gut-healing probiotics.

Positive allergy results are most common during childhood and are often outgrown by adulthood. Food allergy symptoms can be quite subtle and range from gastrointestinal problems, headaches, mood changes, concentration and fatigue. Often people continue to eat these foods, not connecting delayed reactions to foods eaten hours or days before. Elimination of foods that test positive in intolerance or allergy screenings has been found to improve symptoms related to ADHD and Autism.

Sarah has since written to me to inform me that she noticed an immediate behavioural change when Lucas came home from a party one evening having eaten pizza, orange-flavoured drinks containing food additives and other high-sugar foods that he had been avoiding up until then. She described his behaviour as having 'lost complete control', as if he were 'intoxicated'. It is, of course, extremely difficult to control what your children are given at parties, and it is pretty concerning to observe the effects after a period of elimination.

Robyn Silber, Computer Scientist, Software Engineer, ADHD/ASD Advocate

When I was 14, I was diagnosed with ADHD. Ever since then, I've been treating it with medication. From that point forward, I also began receiving disability accommodations in school.

In contrast to high school (secondary school in the UK), dealing with my disability accommodations in college was a nightmare. While I was pursuing my Bachelor of Mathematics, I became so discouraged that I dropped out. It took years of therapy for me to eventually muster up the courage to return to college to finish the degree.

When I returned, I realized that I was going to have to do a lot of self-advocacy. When it came to my accommodations, I'd have to be persistent.

During my first semester back, I found my life calling while taking an intro computer science course in computer programming. I applied to the Master's programme and began the programme a couple of days after earning my Bachelor.

Unfortunately, my professors would try to persuade me from using my accommodations on account of not looking like I had disabilities or because I was the top student in the class.

Near the end of the Master's programme I was diagnosed with Autism Spectrum Disorder. I decided to be open with my professors about it, to raise awareness. Regardless of my openness, my disability accommodations were still not taken seriously. I felt that I was experiencing discrimination.

This difficult time took a toll on my mental health – I suffered from a constant stream of panic attacks, which often impeded me from functioning or taking care of myself.

The good news is I didn't back down and was eventually granted use of my accommodations. I am now a Master of Science in Computer Science and work full-time as a software engineer. I channel the pain from my past as fuel to stand up for myself, stand up for others, and share my story. To anyone who is a parent of a student with disabilities, or works to support a student with disabilities, here are a few words of advice:

- Encourage the student to start self-advocacy early. If a child is still in grade school, have the child participate in her IEP (Individualized Education Plan) meetings. It is important to recognize that accommodations aren't always freely granted to students with disabilities. Even further, if a child has an opinion on her accommodations, it's important that she expresses them. She needs to get into the habit of reflecting on her own disability needs, standing up for herself, and influencing the outcome of her accommodations. In college, this child will be on her own. It will be her responsibility to inform each professor about her accommodations at the start of each semester. Each use of the accommodations in each course requires communicating with the professor. When it comes to timed exams, disability accommodations are often clearly defined. However, in other scenarios, disability accommodations can be a big grey area. She will need to be able to assess these scenarios, determine what accommodations she needs, and ask the professor to grant the accommodations. The more practice a child has with voicing her disability needs, the better prepared she will be to advocate for herself.
- Choose the right college. Do your research. Find a college that has disability services.
- Set up an appointment for your child to meet with a counsellor from the disability centre immediately.

Depending on the school, the disability centre may offer services beyond testing accommodations, such as counselling or help with time management.

- Establish a relationship with someone at the disability centre. Ideally, this person should be someone your child meets with regularly, such as a disability counsellor. Ultimately a child's professors will have the final say in granting use of the accommodations (unless vigorously contested, of course). If the professor is hostile, he or she may discourage or deny your child's use of her accommodations. If this happens, your child's success in finishing school will depend on her relationship with her disability counsellor. It's crucial to have someone influential on your child's team, who is able and willing to advocate on her behalf.
- Persist!

Gregory's Story

Sometimes nutrition is supplemental to medication or just something parents prefer over prescriptions, but even medication doesn't always work. When one intervention doesn't work, you shouldn't give up. I'd like to share with you another client's story where prescriptions could not be used. Gregory's parents contacted me with concerns about their teenage son, Gregory, who had been suffering with inattentive symptoms related to ADD, and some oppositional behaviours at home. His mother explained that Gregory struggled to concentrate (during school, and homework in particular) and was frequently absent-minded and unable to self-motivate. Gregory's parents were primarily interested in a nutritional evaluation as they had previously tried medication but had been forced to discontinue due to its side effects.

My first impressions of Gregory were that he was an extremely polite and well-mannered young man, smart and articulate. He told me that he struggled to pay attention, especially at school, and at home spent a fair amount of time gaming and browsing the internet. A detailed assessment of his medical history revealed Gregory had taken antibiotics frequently as a child, and he self-reported mood swings and bouts of anger and irritability. To our surprise, Gregory's lab results revealed a whopping 38 food intolerances, and seven nutritional insufficiencies in iron, alpha-carotene, zinc, vitamin B2, magnesium and vitamin D, the largest number to date in my observations.

Insufficient levels of magnesium have been observed in children diagnosed with ADHD (Moshfegh *et al.* 2009). Magnesium is required for healthy neurotransmitter function as well as for increasing the production of serotonin receptors (5-HT1A) and helping the calming action of GABA (gamma-aminobutyric acid) (Black *et al.* 2015). Modern processed foods including fizzy drinks (soda), caffeine and white refined sugar can deplete magnesium levels in the body, and insufficient levels can lead to symptoms of irritability, difficulty with concentration, insomnia, depression and anxiety. A small research study which supplemented children with ADHD aged 6–16 with magnesium resulted in a significant improvement in core behavioural symptoms of inattention, impulsivity and hyperactive behaviours, as well as cognitive function (El Baza *et al.* 2016). Other studies have also reported improvements in ADHD symptoms following supplementation with magnesium (Kozielec and Starobrat-Hermelin 1997; Nogovitsina and Levitina 2007). Vitamin B6 also works synergistically to increase magnesium absorption (Mousain-Bosc *et al.* 2004, 2006). Magnesium-rich foods include avocados, bananas, beans and green leafy vegetables.

To increase Gregory's energy levels, I suggested he avoided the processed breakfast cereals he had been eating as these have a high glycaemic load (GL) that result in fluctuations in blood sugar levels (i.e. spikes and dips), with consequences for mood, concentration and attention. I recommended that they tried switching to porridge oats (oatmeal) with a little honey, cinnamon or pureed fruit to flavour, or consider instead preparing a high-protein and omega-3-rich breakfast meal such as vegan (dairy-free) egg whites with an oily fish such as smoked salmon, mackerel, or a vegan omelette with his favourite vegetable fillings.

Due to Gregory's high number of food intolerances, I suggested some nutritional changes to improve his gut microbiome, such as increasing his intake of prebiotic foods (e.g. Jerusalem artichokes, greens, onions, asparagus, bananas and leeks) and supplementing with probiotics. I also suggested a stool test to assess for unhealthy flora. Elevated amounts of antibodies to wheat and gluten are common in the genetic autoimmune condition called *coeliac disease*, and even though most people with elevated antibodies may not test positive for coeliac disease, they may still benefit from the exclusion of these foods from the diet. Coeliac disease is thought to be over-represented in people with ADHD, and a gluten-free diet has improved symptoms of ADHD in those also diagnosed with coeliac disease (Niederhofer 2011).

Gluten and Milk

Studies have shown the beneficial effects of eliminating gluten and cow's milk (switching instead to plant-based alternatives such as flax, coconut or unsweetened hemp milk) in children with ASD and ADHD. The removal of other foods should be guided by the results of an IgG assessment, which will ascertain high, moderate and low intolerances.

Milk intake in autistic children has been found to be linked to constipation and a worsening of general symptoms. Gluten, a protein found in grains such as rye, barley and wheat (including spelt, kamut, farro and durum, and other types such as bulgur and semolina (cream of wheat)), has also been attributed to a worsening of symptoms. Foods high in sugars and/or refined carbohydrates found in white flour, white rice, mashed potatoes and the majority of processed foods have a high GL. These foods drive up blood glucose levels faster than low GL foods, leading to fluctuations in mood, cognition and behaviour. Excessive consumption of high GL foods can lead to insulin resistance, which is one of the first steps in the development of metabolic syndrome, which, in turn, can lead to heart disease, type 2 diabetes and obesity, among other disorders.

Serving slow-release foods for breakfast – such as an omelette, avocado, smoked salmon (lox), porridge oats (oatmeal) or beans – is a great way to keep your child's blood sugar levels stable until lunch. Other examples of low GL foods include oats (rolled or steel-cut), porridge oats (oatmeal), gluten-free muesli (granola), wheat and gluten-free pasta or rice, sweet potato, sweetcorn (corn), yam, butter beans (lima beans), peas, legumes and lentils. Fruits such as cherries, grapefruit, dried apricots, pears, apples, oranges, strawberries, plums and prunes, non-starchy vegetables and carrots are also beneficial.

There is some evidence suggesting that certain gut bacteria may increase the risk of coeliac disease. This is an immune disease that is argued to have appeared after the Neolithic period. It is linked to the introduction of a plethora of dietary changes and increase in food antigens associated with the expansion of agriculture and cereal cultivation. Coeliac disease can also develop in people who are gluten intolerant (Sanz 2010). The behavioural symptoms of coeliac disease are similar to those observed in children diagnosed with ADHD, and so, if your child is diagnosed as having an intolerance to gluten, it is worth testing for (Sanz 2010).

The point I'd like to underline is that diet is modifiable, which means that the discomfort of food intolerances and allergies can be alleviated and may improve behaviour you didn't even realize was a result of an allergy or intolerance.

Chapter Takeaway

- **Allergies are a result of an immune system reaction whereas intolerances are often caused by the lack of a certain enzyme.**
- **Children with ASD and ADHD often experience more food intolerances and allergies than other children.**
- **Milk and gluten are common culprits for allergies or intolerances, and studies have shown that children with ASD and ADHD often benefit from eliminating these items.**
- **Any eliminations should be guided by a screening for allergies and intolerances.**
- **Children with ADHD should be tested for gluten, wheat and diary intolerances at a minimum. A gluten-free diet is considered beneficial to children with ADHD.**

TAKE A STEP

Have an allergy and food intolerance screening done. Consider testing for coeliac disease. Aim for a healthier breakfast that focuses on slow-release foods which can help keep your child's (or your) blood sugar levels stable until lunchtime. You could try porridge (oatmeal), strawberries, oranges, pears, apples, or any of the others named in this chapter.

Chapter 8

Sugars and Dyes

In this chapter I am going to talk about the less healthy foods we eat, even though we might not realize that they are unhealthy, and their potential negative consequences. It is no secret that the food industry has formulated just the right chemical concoctions of sweet (sugar) and savoury (salt) to keep us coming back for more. I often tell children that if you washed the chemical mix off that crisp or chip you are eating, it would taste like cardboard. It would no longer be palatable and you would likely spit it straight back out. The infiltration of junk food can be seen in every Westernized city, and there is no population more vulnerable than children who are brainwashed into thinking these types of processed sugary foods are the norm! Another major factor is that they have not only riddled our societies but are also considered to be addictive as they activate the same reward circuits in the brain as illegal drugs. Increasingly sugar found in processed junk foods is the 'drug' of choice. For us adults, long hours of intense work followed by after-work social engagements can often result in binge drinking, a lack of sleep and then the consumption of unhealthy processed foods as both a comfort and aid to recover.

As I've already detailed, there are strong links between the gut, the brain and the immune system, and high intakes of refined sugar and carbohydrates can promote an unhealthy gut-flora balance, providing the 'fodder' for unhealthy bacteria and yeasts that are known to compromise digestive and immune health (Spangler *et al.* 2004). High sugar levels are also thought to compromise brain function by reducing the 'brain-derived neurotrophic factor', or BDNF, a substance critical for the growth and connectivity of brain cells, as well as for memory and learning. Our old friend the hippocampus is one of only two areas of the brain where adult neurogenesis – the formation of brain cells – takes place. The process is hindered by high levels of saturated fat and refined sugar, which compromise hippocampal activity and affect healthy brain function (Molteni *et al.* 2002).

Sugar is a topic close to the heart of Dr Robert Lustig, Professor of Paediatrics at the University of California, San Francisco, USA. He has described it as the alcohol of the child and explained that the reason we consume so much sugar is quite simply because it is addictive due to its dopamine-releasing abilities. Furthermore, the food industries are well aware of this and know that by adding fructose to everything, the consumer will keep coming back for more (Lustig 2012). Professor Lustig explains that there are five tastes on your tongue: sweet, salty, sour, bitter and savoury (umami). Sugar masks the other four, so you can't taste the negative aspects of foods. He further concludes that even coating a scoop of dog poop in sugar would make it taste good. Can you imagine that?!

What is important to remember here is that *we have no dietary need for manufactured sugars*. Neuroimaging studies have demonstrated that drugs abused by humans activate areas in the ventral striatum – also known as the reward hub of the brain. There is a heated debate among expert scientists that white refined sugar is as addictive as illegal drugs, and yet it is given to children as young as two and three as 'rewards'.

Mike Pickets, Founder of Raver Tots

As a child my ADHD was undiagnosed. Back then there wasn't much help or understanding for what I was going through. In the 1990s, the extent of support I was given by my school was an anger management class, which I had difficulty in understanding because I'd spend every day in fits of hysterics laughing at my own ridiculous behaviour.

The only other support I was given was when I was 14 years old, and I was referred externally to a meeting at the children's centre (similar to the Head Start programme in the US). I attended with my parents, and a key worker (I can't recall his exact role) recited a list of all my recent calamities: 'Detained by police for climbing on the roof of the clock tower on Bournemouth Pier; excluded from school for jumping out of a window; hospitalized after taking an ecstasy tablet; banned from Woking shopping centre for throwing mangos at pedestrians...'

The list went on, and all I can remember doing is laughing uncontrollably while everyone in the room sat and stared at me despondently.

I started to suffer with anxiety and began drinking every day as a coping mechanism. As a 14-year-old boy, I was completely unaware of the term 'anxiety' or its meaning. I used to call it 'paranoia'.

I left school with very few qualifications and was then forced to leave college within a year to work in a series of unstable jobs, often getting fired for bizarre reasons such as throwing telephone sets out of windows, turning up drunk, and on one occasion, hiding a raw fish in my line manager's car bonnet next to his air conditioning unit. Over time, in my twenties, this translated into unstable and dysfunctional relationships.

I became determined to work for myself, as I struggled with directive management (or any management, for that matter), and the structure of a nine-to-five. However, setting up businesses had significant flaws that I'd often overlook. I was often drawn in by my impulsivity and the excitement of taking a risk. I'd often lose money, and I had a string of upset customers when things didn't go to plan. At one stage I even had a disgruntled client throttle me in my office due to an embarrassing misunderstanding.

At the age of 26, I found out I was going to be a dad. It was time to straighten things up, but after several appointments over the years with as little as six counselling sessions to show from it (which were now apparently going to be offered online rather than face to face), I decided to see a private psychiatrist. I was diagnosed with adult ADHD, which came as a bit of a surprise, but also made so much sense.

I began working on a very structured plan to enable me to turn things around. I was given a lot of autonomy in making these plans because of my struggle with authority. The first change was to go completely teetotal (I have now been teetotal for over three years). My next step was to exercise regularly. Within six months I'd focused my energy and addictive personality into running and benefited from the release of endorphins it gave me.

I'd gone from being unable to run to the end of the street to running two marathons. Alongside this came the fine-tuning of my diet, and I suddenly found my life was getting better. My son had been born, followed by my second, and even though I was not living with the mother of my children, through diet, exercise, staying sober and working to a plan, I'd managed to deal with the whole break-up process without any problems and we remain great friends today, sharing equal parenting time with our two young children.

After being persistent in the desire to run my own business over the years, I finally managed to break the formula when I was 29 with my latest company, Raver Tots. I have organically grown a national events business that operates in over 30 cities with over 2000 customers a week in attendance across the nation. The events, where parents can take their children raving in the daytime, made headline news on the BBC, and within the first six months of launching, the videos were viewed over 9 million times.

I often think back to what my music teacher wrote in my yearbook: 'Good luck Michael, you are going to need it.'

The main thing I have learned about having ADHD is that you focus so much on an area of your life that excites you and gives you a high, whether it's good or bad. You can be prone to addiction, and that could mean substances like drugs and alcohol, or positive activities like running and working on a project you love.

The advice I will give my children is to do what makes you happy with your life. I spent years not fitting in, with work, education and relationships. I had a behavioural difference. I didn't learn in the same way as others, and my life is a far cry from the stereotypical two-point-four-children family. But I like it that way and have found a way of seeing the positive sides of ADHD and using them to my advantage.

I hope that this will help anyone reading this to see things in the same light as I do. ADHD is not always a bad thing. It has its challenges, but it can be a really good thing, too, if you focus your energetic and passionate nature into positive things in your life, things that make you happy and things that benefit your own health and wellbeing.

Carly and Connor

Most of my clients have approached me first and foremost because their child is experiencing problems at school, either with symptoms directly or indirectly related to their undiagnosed problems: for example, a failure to thrive, difficulties paying attention, completing school and homework, difficulties following task-related instructions, organization or impulsive behaviours. Let's take Carly and her son Connor as an example.

Carly first approached me as the primary school her son had attended since nursery was threatening to exclude him. She explained that she had struggled on and off for around seven years – having to attend countless school meetings and engage in behaviour interventions that hadn't worked, and his behaviour and self-esteem had spiralled out of control. She felt that she was the only one fighting his corner, and even family and close friends didn't understand him.

Carly is a hard-working, intelligent, single mum of two, and during that initial call she felt she was pretty much out of options and was emotionally drained by the enormity of the situation. I had an immediate two-hour consultation with Carly and Connor, and I outlined ways in which I might be able to help. After meeting with them both, I found Connor to be delightful. But it was clear that he was very unhappy at school, he felt singled out and was frequently getting into trouble and having emotional meltdowns. I carried out some preliminary assessments that included some behaviour checklists and a brief assessment of his verbal and non-verbal reasoning skills.

I had asked Carly to complete a three-day food diary for Connor to better understand the types of foods he was currently eating. With permission from Carly, I also approached his school to arrange a visit to meet with his teachers and the head teacher. During my visit, it was clear that Connor was highly distracted and struggled to retain information and keep up with schoolwork. The pressure of this was causing him anxiety and resulting in emotional outbursts that even his class teacher struggled to soothe. It was clear to me that Connor needed an immediate assessment of these underlying difficulties, and so I made referrals to professionals in my network, including a child and adolescent psychiatrist and a clinical psychologist. Following an in-depth assessment, Connor received diagnoses of ADHD, anxiety and Dyslexia – this explained a lot! Connor had 'survived' (barely) up until this point but was not 'thriving'. His behaviour at school had deteriorated and he had been facing expulsion.

We agreed to start a nutrition plan, and Connor and I chatted about different types of food and how they could positively or negatively affect his moods and behaviour. We agreed for Connor to start taking omega-3 oils, cut out sugar and restrict all refined, processed foods. Connor was keen to learn and incredibly engaging. He was fascinated to learn about sugar and how large intakes at breakfast would create spikes and dips in his blood sugar levels, which would make him feel cranky and affect his concentration, attention and overall energy levels. We agreed to cut out all refined sugar for a while and to choose natural alternatives instead, such as raw honey and cacao, in addition to avoiding all processed foods.

Connor agreed to help his mum with the shopping and his mum even reported that he would enquire at the supermarket if the beef was organic and grass-fed, with no dyes or hormones! At home, Connor agreed to work to improve his omega-3 levels and to take additional mineral and vitamin supplements.

Connor and his mum noticed a difference in just a few weeks of starting the new plan, and one day his teacher called his mum to say that he had been an absolute pleasure in school – something she had never heard before, ever! Connor was relieved to receive his diagnoses and does not view it negatively at all – he explained to me that lots of famous people have ADHD and Dyslexia, and so it is a positive thing to be different! Today, Connor has transitioned into secondary school and has a great group of friends. Carly feels that without the proper investigation of the underlying conditions, change of diet and additional support they would have faced a very different path altogether. And although life is not perfect, they are both much happier.

Food Additives

Food additives are purposefully added to food to preserve shelf life and to alter their appearance, flavour and/or texture (Watts 2008). The EFSA is responsible for food safely in the EU (which the UK may or may not be a part of in the not so distant future). The EFSA has assigned an E number to food additives (synthetic or natural) that have been cleared following safety testing and evaluation into the following classification system:

- E100–E199: Colours.
- E200–E299: Preservatives.
- E300–E399: Antioxidants.
- E400 upwards: Miscellaneous or others.

Food colourings (dyes) and preservatives that are linked to increases in hyperactive behaviour in some children include:

- Sodium benzoate (E211), or sunset yellow, found in jelly, jams, hot chocolate and even infant medicines.
- Quinoline yellow, found in ice cream and lollipops (popsicles).
- Tartrazine, found in soda or fizzy drinks, sweets (candy), chewing gum and yoghurt.
- Allura red, found in sweets (candy), drinks and medicines.

Many European countries, including the UK, have either banned the use of artificial dyes from their food products or require clear labelling as to the type of additive and its purpose in the food. This is in contrast to the FDA in the US, which only requires labelling of FD&C Yellow No. 5 on food packaging. Yellow 6 is used in abundance in the US and can be found in most brands of margarine and even in multivitamin supplements. Other food additives include emulsifiers, flavour enhancers, preservatives such as sulphite, gelling, thickening and stabilizing agents, acids and sweeteners.

A general rule is, if you don't understand the ingredients, put the item back on the shelf! As parents, we have the right to know the effects of processed foods and fizzy drinks (soda) on the brain and body in order to better understand food labels and make valid judgements about the types of foods and beverages to purchase for our families.

Chiltern Way Academy (CWA) Trust

Chiltern Way Academy (CWA) is an award-winning SEN academy for boys and girls aged 9–19 with Autistic Spectrum Condition (ASC), Social, Emotional and Mental Health (SEMH) and Speech Communication and Language Needs (SLCN). Many of our young people have multiple needs sitting beneath these three primary diagnoses, and ADHD is the most prevalent.

Our purpose is to make an enduring difference to our young people's lives, providing them with the knowledge, resilience and skills to enable them to have meaningful and lasting employment. We use every means at our disposal to ensure that this happens.

We are intuitively aware of the impact food has on the students' wellbeing; consequently food has always played an important part in our school life. The students get a high-quality breakfast and a two-course lunch from our in-house catering teams, freshly prepared each day. Our vocational curriculum is dominated by food technology, with many students going on to work in the catering industry.

We are planning a nutritional education and intervention pilot study with Rachel and her team of registered nutritionists. This is not only an exciting opportunity to better understand the role of food in cognitive processing, but also an opportunity for us to use this knowledge to further improve outcomes for our young people.

My son's great success with increasing his omega-3 intake was the catalyst for a series of changes. We enrolled in an organization called the New Learning Centre,[1] founded by Noel Janis-Norton (since changed to the Calmer, Easier, Happier Parenting Centre) in London, which provided a retraining programme in an educational setting for my son during the day and parenting classes for me in the evening. With their guidance, we started an elimination diet, removing all processed and sugar-loaded foods from his diet, and the magic began. It was hard work, especially preparing packed lunches for school, but it had noticeable effects. My son felt ready to try after-school activities once more, choosing acting and boxing, and joined an athletics club, all of which he excelled at.

Food products that may aggravate gut conditions and compromise immunity include sugar, processed carbohydrates and refined foods (e.g. white bread, white pasta and white rice), chemically modified oils and fats (e.g. margarine and refined vegetable oils – try extra virgin cold-pressed olive oil or non-hydrogenated coconut oil instead), and processed meats (e.g. ham and turkey). Adults and children with ADHD should steer away from chemicals in home cleaning products too (opt instead for natural, ecologically friendly cleaning products such as the Method range, Seventh

1 http://calmerparenting.co.uk

Generation, Ecover or Earth Friendly Products). Also consider avoiding fluoride-containing products (e.g. most toothpastes – try natural brands instead, such as Jason's) and avoid antibiotics unless, of course, absolutely necessary, as advised by your medical practitioner. But if you're looking for a one-step-at-a time approach, start by restricting or eliminating white sugar from your or your children's diets. It is arguably one of the worst culprits.

As noted in the study described in Chapter 3, where children were given beverages containing additives and artificial colours (McCann *et al.* 2007), even children without ADHD exhibit ADHD-like symptoms when exposed to these additives and artificial colours. Imagine how much worse it can be for a hyperactive child with ADHD. You may also recall Dr Feingold's testing that found removing food additives caused nearly half of children with ADHD to return to normal behaviour (Feingold 1975). Subsequent replications of Dr Feingold's study revealed the same results. This means all children can benefit from cutting out these food additives.

Chapter Takeaway

- **Sugar is considered by experts such as Professor Robert Lustig as addictive as it activates the same reward circuits in the brain as drugs.**
- **High sugar levels are thought to reduce BDNF, a substance in the brain that is vital for memory, learning and the growth and connectivity of brain cells.**
- **Several food dyes and preservatives are linked to increases in hyperactive behaviour: sodium benzoate, quinoline yellow, tartrazine and Allura Red.**
- **Even children without ADHD can benefit from cutting out additives and dyes from their food.**

TAKE A STEP

Start reading food labels if you don't already do so. Watch out for additives and dyes, and try to eliminate them from your family's diet. Start by cutting out white, refined sugar, especially at breakfast.

Chapter 9

Diets that Help and Diets that Hinder

The world is already full of dietary plans and often dietary advice is out of date and arguably misleading. In this chapter, we are going to take a fresh look at a few common diet types and discover foods which are helpful versus those which research has suggested are not. Knowing which diets suit your family's nutritional needs can help you stock up on recipes when you want something beyond those included at the end of this book.

The Standard American Diet (SAD)

Many children in the West are living on a staple diet of pizza, French fries (chips), chicken tenders (chicken nuggets) and soda (fizzy drinks), commonly known as SAD, or the Standard American Diet. All the while, their brains are being starved of essential fatty acids, vitamins and minerals. Children are arguably the most vulnerable in relation to the SAD; they are over-exposed to processed and refined foods, saturated fats, elevated intakes of sodium, sugar, artificial additives, preservatives and chemicals during critical periods of brain development. In many Western societies, foods have become fast and convenient, manufactured in favour of profit, mass production and shelf life. Sadly, somewhere along the way, the food industry has lost sight of the fact that nutritional content should be the focal point. Many consumers do not fully understand food labels and artificial ingredients such as *high-fructose corn syrup (HFCS)* or *hydrogenated soybean oil*, or the harms that can arise from the habitual consumption of processed foods.

In terms of nutrition, the Western diet or SAD can be characterized as having a high sodium content; a low nutrient density in relation to the amount of minerals, vitamins and trace elements, antioxidants, fibre, phytochemicals, amino acids and unsaturated fatty acids per gram; and a high GL due to the presence of refined sugars and grain products. This has led the United Nations (UN) to acknowledge a new type of malnutrition, coined 'Type B', arguably the result of multiple micronutrient depletion and the globalization of our Western food systems.

Moreover, the 21st century has witnessed not only the introduction of a prolific number of chemicals in our environment, but also an abundance of new constituents in foods. These include the global use of pesticides and fertilizers as opposed to crops developing and growing (or animals grazing) in a natural environment. There is also a high concentration of saturated fats from fatty domestic meats, as opposed to wild mammals that arguably contain higher protein and heart-healthy LC-PUFAs (Strazdiņa, Jemeļjanov and Sterna 2013).

Junk Food as a Reward

You can expect most modern diets to provide a laundry list of artificial additives, chemicals, colours and preservatives. Such well-thought-out chemical concoctions! These types of foods are grabbed for their purported convenience, taste and price, and children, unfortunately, are one of the most vulnerable groups because they are frequently 'treated' or 'rewarded' with a plethora of junk food: trips to McDonalds and confectionery treats given on celebratory occasions such as birthdays, Easter and Christmas. Sugar has become an integral part of children's lives in the same way as the consumption of alcohol by adults. By allowing more than the occasional binge in sugar and other refined food substances we are increasing the risk of problem eating behaviours and the development of life-long addictions.

Think about what your child might eat at a conventional birthday party. Will it be fresh fruit, hummus and vegetable crudités? Or is it more likely to be crisps (chips), chocolate cake and white bread with processed meat sandwiches and fizzy drinks (soda)? Any parent observing their child devour the latter menu will know instinctively the consequences of junk food on their child's behaviour. This was the premise of a mock party stunt I helped Betty TV stage in 2012 during an episode of Channel 4's *The Food Hospital* programme.

We staged a party in a village town hall for approximately 80 primary school children aged six to eight. The room was divided into two teams, red and blue. The blue team was assigned to the healthy tea party group (sandwiches, fruit, carrot sticks, hummus, homemade fish fingers (fish sticks) and chicken goujons) while the red team was presented with traditional party junk food such as Party Rings (a type of cookie), Haribo sweets (candy), cakes, chocolate, lollies, sausage rolls and crisps (chips). After eating, the children participated in organized games such as 'musical chairs' and 'pass the parcel'. A group of psychologists rated their behaviour, recording the number of aggressive incidents (pushes, tantrums, shouting, etc.).

It came as no surprise to observe the junk food party children acting up very quickly. We witnessed karate kicks, temper tantrums, crying, hyperactivity, and more. Needless to say, the red team won hands down for the highest ratings of aggressive incidents compared to the blue team.

The Ketogenic Diet

This diet featured heavily in the popular (and controversial) Netflix documentary *The Magic Pill*. If you haven't already watched it, I suggest you do. It was filmed in the US and Australia and followed several families suffering with chronic ill health and one little girl with fairly severe Autism. The intervention was the ketogenic (keto) diet, and after 10 weeks all the families reported marked and visible improvements. The little girl became more sociable; she even said her first word and was seen holding a fork as opposed to eating with her hands. She had fewer seizures, and her parents were even able to start weaning her off the anti-convulsant narcotic drugs she was on. So, what is the keto diet, you might be wondering? Well, it is a high-fat, low-protein, low-carbohydrate diet, and has been used medically to manage seizures in children with epilepsy. The exact mechanism of this diet is unclear, but it is related to the negative balance of sodium and potassium that the diet implements.

A study conducted by Pulsifer *et al.* (2001) tested the ketogenic diet in 65 epileptic children attending Johns Hopkins Medical Hospital in the US. The children, aged between 18 months to 14 years 6 months, were tested before starting the diet and at a one-year follow-up. The results demonstratively reduced seizures and the need for antiepileptic medication, and resulted in an increase in overall developmental functioning, especially in the motor skills. There were also significant differences in attention and social functioning. Seizures had been reduced from 25 per day to less than 2 a day at the year follow-up. There is a sizeable overlap between epilepsy and symptoms of ADHD and Autism, and so there is an argument to support the notion that this diet may also benefit these groups. Emerging evidence also suggests it may be beneficial for a wide range of diseases including cardiovascular disease, diabetes and cancer.

The diet advises:

- Limiting to foods that are high in healthy fat content (olive and coconut oils, wild fish and seafood, free-range meats, eggs and avocado), low in protein content and low in carbohydrate content.

- Eliminating all processed foods.
- Avoiding vegetable oils.
- Introducing organic bone broths, organic meat, fermented foods and intermittent fasting.
- Eating whole and organic foods.

You can see that some of these recommendations overlap with suggestions already made in this book.

The Feingold Diet

You may recall Dr Feingold from Chapters 3 and 8. Dr Feingold found that modifying a child's diet and restricting the intake of artificial flavours and colours resulted in a 60–70 per cent decrease of behavioural issues in children with disturbances. While his work has been subjected to criticism because it was based on case studies and not randomized controlled trials, it has since been an influential landmark in the field of nutrition and neurodevelopmental disorders. Here are the ingredients he suggests avoiding:

- Dyes, such as Red 3, Red 40, Blue 1, Blue 2, Yellow 5, Yellow 6, Green 3, Yellow 10, Red 30, and others.
- Artificial flavours, such as vanillin.
- Artificial sweeteners, such as aspartame (contained in brands such as NutraSweet and Equal) and sucralose (e.g. Splenda).
- Preservatives, such as BHA, BHT and TBHQ (petrochemicals, made from petroleum and not allowed in some countries).

Veganism and Omega-3s

I am often asked, 'What if I am vegan and choose not to eat fish, seafood, omega-3-rich eggs or grass-fed meats, how can I obtain my omega-3s?' The answer, bluntly, is 'not easily'.

As already mentioned, the main form of plant-based omega-3 is the short-chain polyunsaturated fatty acid (SC-PUFA) alpha-linolenic acid (ALA). ALA can be obtained by eating certain nuts (such as walnuts), seeds (such as pumpkin seeds or flax seeds) and green leafy vegetables such as kale, or algae such as spirulina. Small amounts may also be found in spinach, Brussels sprouts, eggs, and for non-vegans, meat from cows and sheep that have been grass-fed. However, the biochemical conversion of SC-PUFAs into the LC-HUFAs your brain needs – EPA and DHA – is problematic and mediated by a multitude of factors such as age, genetics, whether you are male or female, your background diet (i.e. what you normally eat) and whether or not you smoke cigarettes and/or drink alcohol.

If you are only eating plant-based forms of ALA, you will need to substantially increase your intake to optimize the probability of bodily conversion into the LC-HUFAs. In this instance, you may wish to try supplementing with an algae-derived DHA capsule (readily available in online health food stores). You should also conduct the omega-3 finger-prick test every three months or so to make sure you're hitting the optimal levels.

The Mediterranean Diet

We've already discussed the known benefits of the Mediterranean diet, namely, that those who ascribe to this diet have lower rates of ADHD and/or its symptoms. In Chapter 3, it was mentioned that this diet is linked to a longer life span and lower rates of many diseases, including mental illnesses. This diet consists of lean meat, olive oil, nuts and seeds, salad leaves, vegetables, and fish and seafood. From Chapter 5, we know how beneficial oily fish and seafood can be.

The Pescatarian Diet

This diet resembles the Mediterranean diet, and consists of fruit, vegetables, lots of green leafy vegetables, nuts, seeds, olive oil and fish. There is so much variety of fish and seafood. Some of my own favourites include: grilled sardines, sea bass, trout, salmon, snapper, Dover sole, scallops, squid and king prawn shrimp (see the recipes at the end of the book). If you are worried about the risk of mercury contamination, avoid shark, swordfish, marlin, orange roughy, ahi tuna and tilefish, and choose instead wild-caught produce from a local fishmonger.

Perhaps your family already uses one of these diet plans, but maybe not. Either way, the cookbooks for some of these diets could be helpful in revamping your nutrition plan. Your teenager will inevitably be lured away by pizzas and burgers to a certain degree, but you can offset the problem by keeping the food consistently healthy at home. If you've spent years helping them 'acquire a taste' for fish and other good stuff, please don't give up!

Chapter Takeaway

- **The typical Western diet relies on fast, easy food that is loaded with additives, dyes and sugar.**
- **The Mediterranean diet (along with others) places a focus on fresh vegetables and wild fish, which correlate to lower rates of disease.**
- **Know that your child will not always stick to the diet you set, but setting an example by implementing it for all the family and eating together at home is important.**

TAKE A STEP

Buy a new cookbook or source some recipes from the internet for a collection that focuses on all the healthy and enjoyable food items you want in your family's diet. Try searching for Mediterranean recipes or cookbooks. It's important to amass a variety of recipes to avoid boredom.

Chapter 10

Eating Mindfully

We all live in a fast-paced, digital, consumer-oriented world where everything is replaceable. It can feel as if we are exposed to a conveyor belt of choices that creates confusion and leaves us vulnerable to making careless, impulsive and self-serving decisions – like consuming quick, poor-quality food and self-medicating on substances such as excessive alcohol – which, in turn, negatively influences our commitment to change, our ability to be responsible, and our relationships.

Whether you're reading this as a practitioner or a parent, you can decide to make a change to your diet or a child's diet. Deciding on a new path is the first step, but there's more to it than just *knowing* what's best. Mindfulness is growing quite popular these days, and applies to many different facets of life. In this chapter, I look at how we can apply the principles of mindfulness to nutrition and feeding our bodies and our children's bodies.

Eating Mindfully

Healthy eating does not immediately come naturally to many

people. It has to be learned, and then acquired mindfully to create an inner awareness of clean and conscious eating. The great news is that it is never too late to start, and you can congratulate yourself for picking up a copy of this book and being committed to start the process, and to supporting those around you or those you work with to do the same. If you make this change personally, your future self will thank you for it, as you optimize your family's physical and mental health.

No one else can do this for an individual. We can guide other people, but ultimately, it is the individual, in the end, who is responsible for making changes. So encourage yourself and those around you. Anyone wishing to make long-lasting and mindful changes to their diet needs to be their own best friend and go easy on themself along the way.

There are no expectations to get it right immediately, but the journey starts by making the decision to change and taking action every single day. Remind yourself or those you work with that it is important to embrace and enjoy the commitment to change and have fun finding creative ways that work for you and your family. This is the single greatest investment in life you can make.

Adopting a mindful approach translates to understanding that choosing a home-cooked, fish-based meal over a frozen pizza is a small change in the direction towards health and wellness. You, or those you work with, will find that within just a short space of time this new habit will become embedded into daily behaviour, and the old pattern of thinking 'I'll just grab a pizza' rapidly fades away. This process is called neuroplasticity – pathways in the brain will become redundant and will eventually be pruned away, and new synapses will grow in their place, reinforcing the new behaviour. This is the exciting process of rewiring your brain!

There are various theories about how long it takes to change a habit, from 21 days to two months or longer. The single one thing you should remember is this – the brain is a remarkable organ, capable of regenerating new cells and pathways via neuroplasticity. Connections in the brain can either strengthen or weaken according to the brain's activity and functions. Keeping this in mind, the best way to create a new habit, or encourage those you work with to do so, is by practising it one day at a time. Yup, rote learning really does work. The process of repetition is a simple formula: make a decision, act on it, and repeat! This formula, one day at a time, is error-proof. The acquisition of new skills has been clinically demonstrated to alter both the structure and function of our brains – encourage the children you support to imagine that. We are capable of changing our brain. This exciting concept is both empowering and uplifting. So, for the purposes of creating change, I will ask you, and those you work with, to keep in mind that the first 28 days of any concentrated change programme is sufficient to re-set your mind state, to re-energize and to re-educate yourself.

The secret, in my opinion, to improving an individual's life and health and changing old, redundant habits that no longer serve them well is simply to take affirmative action and repeat it every day; it is as simple as that. Taking some steps every day towards changing old habits means over time you will have created new ways of thinking, being and doing. The acquisition of new skills therefore requires persistence and repetition.

What is critically important is that an individual takes a mindful approach across multiple domains of their life, and I invite you to now evaluate these in relation to your current situation. The five domains include: psychological (e.g. thoughts, feelings, actions and everyday behaviour), biological (which includes the maintenance of your bodily systems and the healthy functioning of your brain), nutritional (which, it goes without saying, I believe is critical for everything!), physical (e.g. how much exercise you are taking daily, taking care of your body and skin) and, of course, practising *self-love*. There are many resources out there on how mindfulness in all of these areas can improve one's state of being.

The practice of mindful meditation has been found to be helpful for children; it can encourage them to listen and communicate more thoughtfully as well as support emotional reactivity. Several studies have found mindfulness to be especially useful to individuals with ADHD.[1]

Make a Plan: Meal Planning Charts

It's time to make a simple plan so you can start implementing changes. Grab a pencil (this is important, so you can erase and update things as you adopt new nutritional habits), as I would like you to complete a little daily exercise for 28 days. You can use it as a meal planning chart or just a way to track how your changes are progressing. You might choose to include any changes you observe in your child's behaviour in relation to what you do differently food-wise. This could help you observe trends in which foods may alleviate your child's symptoms.

Keeping a record of the small positive changes you are making daily will help you track how things change. Small steps in this direction daily add up to significant changes over time, which you and your child will be grateful for.

Aside from everything else we've discussed in this book, there are some other ways you could implement mindful changes in your family's environment.

---

1 See www.uclahealth.org/marc/research.

Day	Nutritional changes Week 1	Nutritional changes Week 2	Nutritional changes Week 3	Nutritional changes Week 4	Nutritional changes Week 5
Monday	Made a juice (60% veg and 40% low GI fruit) for breakfast				
Tuesday	Cut out bread and opted for a salad + protein lunch instead				
Wednesday	Cooked a meal from scratch, using healthy, organic produce				
Thursday	Cut out sugar for 24 hours				
Friday	Drank 2l of alkaline water				
Saturday	Invested in healthy spices and herbs to cook with. Took omega-3 oils and multivitamin				
Sunday	Added probiotics to shopping list				

Think about the Dishes

In order to avoid possible exposure to toxins, and to also choose cooking equipment that is environmentally friendly, I have created a list of my personal preferences to guide you, or those you work with, in cooking mindfully:

- Consider avoiding aluminium (aluminum), Teflon and plastic.
- Consider eco-friendly cookware such as clay, bamboo, cast iron, glass (e.g. Pyrex) or ceramic (e.g. non-stick coating that is PTFE, PFOA and cadmium free).
- If you are using stainless steel, be mindful that if the food you are cooking is too acidic, there is a possibility the pan may leak chromium, cobalt and nickel into the food, so if adults or children are allergic to nickel be careful, as stainless steel can cause reactions.
- If using plastic containers for storage, I advise choosing BPA-free plastic or use glass instead. When heated, plastic may release chemicals called dioxins into foods that are thought to be potentially harmful.
- I personally choose not to use microwaves as I prefer that all meals be made from scratch and be freshly prepared. Be aware that when using microwaves, food wrapped in plastic or plastic containers may leak BPA and phthalates into your food. These are referred to as endocrine disrupters due to their ability to mimic human hormones. Look out for the 'microwave safe' label if in doubt.

Hydrate

People often overlook the importance of staying hydrated. They may simply forget to drink or don't realize they are thirsty. Symptoms of dehydration can be mild to moderate, and can range from headaches to dry skin, a dry or sticky mouth and muscle cramps (Cheuvront and Kenefick 2014). The simplest way of establishing whether or not someone is dehydrated is to check the colour of their urine. If it is dark yellow or brown, they are dehydrated. Severe dehydration can lead to confusion, irritability, anxiety, a rapid heartbeat and breathing, lack of energy, sunken eyes, feeling dizzy and fainting.

Excessive exercise, diarrhoea, vomiting, excessive sweating, too much sun and diseases or conditions like diabetes or severe sun burn all cause dehydration. Flying is also thought to increase the risk of dehydration, so take precautions for any trip and hydrate adequately afterwards.

Our bodily composition is around two-thirds water, which fills all the cells in our bodily tissue, and importantly, is critical for brain function. Water delivers nutrients to the brain and removes toxins. An inadequate daily intake of water will affect an individual's cognitive performance, concentration, thought processing and alertness, so be sure to drink around eight glasses of filtered or mineral water every day. This is a must – not only will it fully hydrate you, it will also promote weight loss, and improve your skin, attention and focus. I personally carry a 2-litre bottle around with me that I sip from during the day to ensure I am getting my day's supply.

Timing of Meals

Make sure that the last meal of the day is not too late in the evening or close to bedtime, especially for children. Instead, if hungry, consider a light, low-glycaemic complex carbohydrate snack (try a small amount of cherries, peach slices, a bowl of porridge (oatmeal), a slice of wholegrain pumpernickel toast with peanut butter or hummus or a small portion of sweet potato mash instead, to keep hunger at bay.

Robert Picardo, Actor and Advocate of Brain Health

As an actor, I have had the opportunity to play a broad range of characters and to work with an even broader range of people. The considerable overlap in the Venn diagram for the creative personality and the ADHD personality has been evident throughout my training as an actor and my 40+ years as a working professional. When I am at my best creatively, I am recognizably – and proudly – 'on the spectrum', although I emphasize that this is only a self-diagnosis (and from a former TV doctor at that!).

For many years, I played a future medical technology on television: the Emergency Medical Hologram in *Star Trek: Voyager*. Although my character was an advanced artificial intelligence programmed with everything we know about medicine in the 24th century, he was primarily a new technology with recurring software issues. His emotional subroutines ('bedside manner') needed an upgrade. There were also a number of episodes in which technical issues with his program mimicked human brain or neurological disorders, so that our writers could examine the challenges – on the individual and crew mates ('loved ones') – of Alzheimer's disease (my memory engrams are decompiling!), nervous breakdown (in choosing to save one critically injured crew member over another, I develop a recurrent conflict in my Hippocratic Oath subprogram!), amnesia (my system reboots to 'factory issue' parameters!), psychopathy/personality disorder (upgrading my program with qualities from historical figures creates a Mr Hyde-like alter ego!), and uncontrollable hallucination (expanding my program to include the capacity to 'daydream' like my organic colleagues renders me incapable of distinguishing between fantasy and reality!), to name a few.

In sum, if my experiences as a 24th-century medical professional on *Star Trek* have taught me anything, it's that we need to increase our passion to look both inside and beyond ourselves. Our brains and our universe are the endless frontiers of life-enhancing discovery.

The take-home message around mindful eating is to take small positive steps every day, which your future self will thank you for.

Chapter Takeaway

- **The brain's habits can be changed and new pathways formed through neuroplasticity.**
- **Mindfulness in eating means being attentive to unhelpful and unhealthy food habits that urge you to take the easy way.**
- **Each day and every day, make a choice to stick with one beneficial change for the better health of your family; over time the practice of this new habit will lead to brain-based changes.**
- **Nutrition is a major component of health, but you should use it with other mindfulness practices to attain the best results for your child and your family.**

TAKE A STEP

Use the chart in this chapter and start planning small changes for the next 28 days. You'll form new, healthier habits for your family. Take a look at your kitchenware and see what could be replaced with something eco-friendly and toxin-free.

Conclusion

Well, we have reached the end of this book's journey for now. I trust you have enjoyed reading the rich material provided and will be able to apply it now with positive outcomes for both you and your family, or for those you work with.

The brain really is capable of change, and reading this book is the start of that journey! I do hope you will enjoy preparing the assortment of delicious recipes I have included in the following pages, from friends and associates including celebrity fish and seafood chef Rick Stein, Michelin star chef Tom Kerridge, Randy Hartnell of Vital Choice and my good friend Adrian Luckie, founder of Mama's Jerk.

Nutrition is an undeniable and critical component of health and wellbeing, but it is only a part of the whole process. The key message is that people with ADHD are so much more than the symptoms they present with, and any type of therapeutic intervention must address all aspects of our life (e.g. psychological, biological, social and spiritual – all of which can impact the physical body) in order to heal.

Whether you are a professional or a parent, please remember, being a mum or dad to a child with any type of learning or behaviour difference is extremely challenging. It requires patience, empathy and understanding beyond normal levels. I like to take comfort and remind myself and others that special children are given to special parents – a belief I subscribe to when taking off my scientific hat! The experience is life changing, and in spite of all the challenges thrown at these parents, most learn the language, they cope, and become their own educators.

For all those living with and supporting those with any type of neurodiverse condition, I salute you. I know this journey can be tough, so please congratulate yourself that you have come this far. Sometimes when we feel we are weathering a storm, we just need to pause a little and adjust the sails.

Self-love and self-care will make the biggest difference, and healthy eating is a major part of this process. Above all, we have to be our own best friend if we are to support those around us, and this requires a large dose of self-nurturing and nourishing to reach the final destination of health and complete wellness of body and mind.

If it weren't for my son's diagnosis of ADHD, which took me out of my career comfort zone all those years ago, I wouldn't be on this journey and writing this book today. It has been a rocky road, with many obstacles and roadblocks along the way, but, as the saying goes, *nothing worthwhile in life is easy!*

This book will help with nutrition, but there is much more you can do, too. Never stop seeking ways to support those around you who have ADHD and struggle with mental health to live their best lives and to realize their full potential. I would love to hear how the book has motivated or educated you, so please do get in contact via my website or social media platforms.

Recipes

I have included a selection of recipes here to help optimize brain health, and to assist with the symptoms of ADHD, improving mental function, behaviour and mood.

One of my recipe providers certainly doesn't need further endorsement from me, being one of the most popular British foodies of all time. Christopher Richard 'Rick' Stein CBE is a celebrated fish and seafood chef, author and TV celebrity. My introduction to Rick came from my good friend Professor John Stein, Rick's brother, an eminent neuroscientist and world expert in Dyslexia, who spent a good part of his career at the University of Oxford's Magdalen College. I had the great pleasure of first meeting Rick in 2010 when he agreed to cater for an event I had co-organized in honour of Professor Michael Crawford's 80th birthday. The event was called the 'DHA Celebration Meeting', held at the Royal Society of Medicine in London, and was attended to capacity with scientists arriving from all over the world, all with an interest in the biological and health benefits of healthy and essential omega-3 fats.

Another good friend provided me with four recipes: Adrian Luckie, lucky by name and also by nature! Adrian first founded Mama's Jerk in London on 1 March 2009 as a tribute and legacy to his late great-grandmother, Mama Charlotte, who was born and raised in St Elizabeth, Jamaica. Mama's Jerk is in several locations across London, serving up healthy and delicious Caribbean-influenced food for those of us who like a little spice in our life!

Four recipes were kindly shared by a dear friend, Randy Hartnell, founder of Vital Choice, a premium fish and seafood company that delivers fresh produce of the highest quality right to your door! Vital Choice is renowned for its top-quality, sustainably produced wild salmon, wild seafood, organic food and grass-fed meat and poultry. In 2014, the company became a Certified B Corporation, in recognition of its sustainable sourcing and socially responsible practices. Before founding Vital Choice with his wife Carla in 2002,

Washington State native Randy spent more than 20 years fishing wild, pristine Alaskan waters for salmon, herring and other regional species. As Randy says, 'Good health is our most precious gift, and nothing can support or undermine it more than the foods we choose to eat each day. Our mission is to help our customers find and enjoy deeply nourishing "real" foods.' From the beginning, Randy sought out leading scientific experts specializing in the health effects of seafood and omega-3 fatty acids. It is their research that guided and inspired the creation of the recipes included here.

I was also honoured to be invited to cast my scientific eye over the Michelin Star celebrity chef Tom Kerridge's book, *The Dopamine Diet: My Low-Carb, Stay-Happy Way to Lose Weight*. I am even more thrilled to be able to share with you three of my favourite recipes from his book. I hope you enjoy these as much as I do!

Child-Friendly Meals

Many parents have witnessed fussy and restrictive food behaviours in their children, and this is especially the case for many children with Autism and ADHD. There are many theories about why this develops and some preliminary evidence suggests that certain processed foods are promoting the growth of unhealthy gut microbiota that over time may lead to leaky gut syndrome. The ideal scenario is, of course, to get them eating healthy foods right from the start and to avoid altogether processed, refined foods, but hindsight is a great thing! Children with neurodiverse symptoms of ADHD and Autism can be very rigid and inflexible when it comes to eating. It is common for them to gravitate towards what is commonly known as the 'white' foods (i.e. white potatoes, white rice, white pasta, white sugar, chicken nuggets (chicken tenders), and so on). But the good news is that even if your child is already following the 'white' food diet, this can be undone within three to four weeks of persistence, encouragement and rewards (non-food based). For young children, you could create a reward poster with each day marked and a space to place stickers (see my website at drrachelvgow.com, for more information).

Changing nutritional habits is challenging, but the brain does adjust and make modifications when we introduce new habits and persistently repeat them; cravings will eventually lessen and the old behaviour will fade away, with new pathways in the brain emerging. Dr Alex Richardson discusses more about changing nutritional habits in Chapter 11 of her book *They Are What You Feed Them* (2006). To help you get started, I have included some healthy and delicious meals that will give your children's brains a boost they deserve! These recipes are marked as 'child friendly' for reference purposes; however, it is recommended that mealtimes are family-based and the recipes are inclusive to all members. I have also included some recipes that allow for food intolerances to gluten, wheat and diary.

Encourage children into the kitchen, with their own chef's hat and apron, and get them cooking with you! Make mealtimes light-hearted and avoid making food the focus – instead, sit around the table together and chat. The more pressure you put on your children to eat, the more likely food will become an issue. Serve food on your child's favourite plate, and if they are fussy about food groups touching, place vegetables in bright bowls. Teach them about food, their origin and how they help bodies grow and the brain to work to its best. Persistence and repetition are essential with young children – always serve fruit and vegetables so they become normalized. Let them see you eating them and comment on how delicious and healthy they are. Change is never easy but it is entirely within your reach, and the rewards are in the pleasure of seeing your child thrive.

Whole Food Information

- Avocados offer approximately 20 vitamins and minerals in every serving (50g). They contain potassium (helps control blood pressure), lutein (good for the eyes) and folate (crucial for cell repair and during pregnancy). They are also a good source of B vitamins, which can help fight disease and infection. They contain vitamins C and E, as well as natural plant chemicals and are heart-healthy.
- Courgettes (zucchini) are also low in calories and a great source of vitamins A, C and folate.
- Eggs contain selenium, a key nutrient for brain health.
- Garlic has antiviral and antibacterial properties that help prevent or fight infection. Garlic may also prevent certain cancers and lower high blood pressure and elevated blood cholesterol.
- Kale contains vitamin C and is a rich source of beta-carotene. It is also a source of folate, calcium, iron and potassium. It contains bioflavonoids, which can protect against some diseases.
- Peppers (bell peppers) are low in calories (approximately 32kcal per medium-size pepper), and contain vitamin C and beta-carotene.
- Red onions are thought to lower blood pressure and cholesterol, are a good source of vitamin C and beta-carotene and have a mild antibacterial effect.
- Rocket contains calcium, vitamin C, beta-carotene, iron and folate. It is one of the most nutritious salad greens and all for only 16 calories per 100g serving!

- Sirloin steak and lean mince from cows that have been grass-fed is a rich source of protein with a wide-range of nutrients including vitamin B12, iron, niacin and zinc.
- Smoked salmon (lox) contains brain-essential omega-3s that help regulate dopamine and reduce symptoms of depression and ADHD. It is also great for the skin and helps protect against heart disease, diabetes and arthritis. It has been demonstrated to significantly reduce clinical symptoms of both ADHD and depression.
- Sweet potatoes are loaded with phytonutrients, fibre, beta-carotene, vitamins C and B6, folate and potassium.
- Tomatoes contain lycopene, which is protective against some diseases as well as being a great source of vitamin C, potassium, folate and beta-carotene.

Here are some of my favourites dishes that can be enjoyed by children and adults alike. My advice is always to encourage your child and partner to get cooking in the kitchen with you – make it fun and experimental by switching ingredients, there are no rules! Enjoy eating your way to brain health.[1]

---

1 For US conversions of measurements, see, for example, www.convert-me.com/en/convert/cooking.

Breakfast

James Caleb Jackson, a religiously conservative vegetarian, invented the first breakfast cereal in around 1863 as a digestive aid. However, many supermarket cereals now are nothing more than a sugary snack fortified with synthetic chemical additives. My advice for getting healthy is to ditch the breakfast cereals unless homemade, such as muesli with berries (or similar), or prepare from scratch a meal of protein, omega-3 and other healthy brain-essential nutrients.

I recommend starting your day by first drinking a glass of freshly squeezed, vitamin C-loaded lemon or lime juice with filtered or mineral water at room temperature to dilute. Lemon or lime water helps flush out toxins, is immune boosting, aids digestion, improves the skin, freshens the breath and helps promote weight loss. You may wish to drink through an environmentally friendly straw to protect teeth enamel.

Organic Honey, Fruit and Almond Porridge [child-friendly]

SERVES 1

- 30g organic rolled oats (oatmeal)
- 250ml milk (plant-based or A2)
- 20g pureed apple or other fruit (e.g. apricots, fresh or dried, strawberries)
- 2 teaspoons organic ground cinnamon (optional)
- 1 tablespoon ground almonds (or flax seeds) (optional)
- 1 tablespoon raisins (optional)
- 1 tablespoon Manuka honey or raw organic version
- A handful of blueberries (optional)

1 Soak the oats ideally overnight or a few hours beforehand (this helps to break down starches and reduce the naturally occurring phytic acid (the outer layer of all grains) which improves nutrient absorption).

2 Heat the milk over a medium heat and add the pureed apple, ground cinnamon and oats. Cook for about 3 minutes, stirring, until soft.

3 Add the ground almonds and raisins for 1 minute, and gently stir.

4 Check the porridge is the right consistency for you and cooked through. Pour into a serving bowl.

5 Add a drizzle of honey and top with blueberries.

NOTE FOR PARENTS

- Organic rolled oats contain vital nutrients such as B complex vitamins, beta-glucans, manganese, phosphorus, magnesium, copper, iron, zinc and folate. They also contain antioxidants called avenanthramides, which have an anti-inflammatory effect. They are a slow-release food that helps to balance blood sugar levels and will help to keep cognition and mood stable.
- Manuka honey is lower in sugar than other honey, has many health benefits, is antibacterial, and can help soothe sore throats, aid digestion, protect against infections and improve immunity and skin.

Omega-3 Breakfast Bites [child-friendly]

MAKES 18

125g skinless and boneless sardines, pilchards or mackerel (ideally cooked from fresh)

2 tablespoons homemade or vegan natural mayonnaise

⅛ teaspoon turmeric

Ground black pepper or cayenne pepper

2 tablespoons flat-leaf parsley, chopped

Half an organic cucumber

3 sheets of Nori (edible seaweed)

1 Mash the sardines, pilchards or mackerel with a fork in a bowl. Mix in the mayonnaise, turmeric, pepper and parsley.

2 Cut 12 matchsticks, 10cm long, from the half a cucumber, and put to one side. Mash the remaining cucumber into the fish mixture.

3 Place the Nori sheets on a work surface, shiny side facedown. About 2.5cm from the edge of the Nori sheet, spread one-third of the fish mixture over each sheet, leaving about 5cm on the opposite end.

4 Place 4 cucumber matchsticks length-wise across the sardine mixture at the near edge of each Nori sheet, and starting from the edge nearest you, roll tightly into a sushi-style roll.

5 Seal each roll by wetting the seam with water and pressing down firmly. Use a sharp knife to cut each Nori roll into 6 pieces, 2.5cm wide, trim off messy ends if needed, and serve.

Smoked Salmon, Scrambled Eggs and Avocado with a Side of Rocket and Tomatoes

Preparation time for this is around 5 minutes, with a cooking time of around 7 minutes, so it makes a healthy and delicious breakfast meal in around 12 minutes, which will stabilize blood sugar levels and keep you alert, focused and happy until lunchtime.

SERVES 1

2 organic, free-range eggs, beaten

Olive oil

Black pepper

Rocket (arugula) or organic salad leaves

A few slices of smoked salmon (lox)

Half an avocado, crushed with lime juice (optional)

A few tomatoes on the vine, thinly sliced

Balsamic vinegar

1 Pour the eggs into a frying pan with a little olive oil mixed in, add a little black pepper, and scramble.

2 Serve on a bed of rocket or salad leaves.

3 Add the smoked salmon, avocado and tomatoes, with a sprinkling of balsamic vinegar.

Crepes with Dark Chocolate Hazelnut Spread [child-friendly]

This is a real Saturday breakfast treat!

MAKES 8

FOR THE DARK CHOCOLATE HAZELNUT SPREAD:

300g skinless hazelnuts or almonds*

1 tablespoon coconut oil

4 tablespoons raw cacao

75g coconut sugar

FOR THE CREPES:

4 organic, free-range eggs

225ml almond milk

125g buckwheat flour

Unrefined salt (optional)

1 tablespoon coconut oil

3 tablespoons coconut flakes

1 Spread the hazelnuts onto a baking tray and roast at 140°C/Gas Mark 1 for 15–20 minutes, and remove the skins once cooked. Leave to cool.

2 Grind them in a food processor with 1 tablespoon of the coconut oil.

3 Add the raw cacao and coconut sugar. Blend for a further 5–10 minutes, until the texture is smooth.

4 To make the crepes, whisk the eggs and milk in a large bowl, sift in the flour and add a pinch of unrefined salt.

5 Heat 1 tablespoon of coconut oil in a frying pan over a medium heat.

6 Pour in a small amount of the mix, ensuring even distribution across the base of the pan. When the edges start to curl up, flip the crepe over and spoon a small amount of the chocolate hazelnut spread in the middle.

7 Cook for 30 seconds and fold in half. Serve with a sprinkle of coconut flakes.

NOTE

* If your child is intolerant or allergic to nuts, replace the nuts with 140g softened unsalted butter and approximately 60ml water.

Blended Juices and Drinks

I recommend a blended fruit and vegetable juice every morning for at least the first 28 days, and then reduce to two or three times a week. If you have a NutriBullet or a similar blender you can make enough to put in the fridge at work and have a blended juice instead of lunch. These juices really give the brain and body a boost – your entire bodily system is going to be loaded with all the vitamins, fibre and antioxidants it needs to get through the day. Try adding immune-boosting slivers of garlic, ginger, parsley and turmeric.

Nutrient-Rich Smoothie

Here is a list of a few of my favourite fruits and vegetables to blend, but you can also choose your own. Experiment with different versions, but try to aim for a ratio of 60 per cent raw vegetables to 40 per cent fruit (peel, chop and wash the fruit and vegetables first).

Spinach	Celery
Kale	Red grapes
Carrot	Tomatoes
Beetroot (beets)	Watermelon
Blueberries	Strawberries
Nectarine	Pineapple
Mango	

1 Place your choice of fruit and vegetables in a NutriBullet or a similar blender, add filtered or mineral water, blend for a few minutes and then serve.

Carrot, Beetroot and Apple Smoothie [child-friendly]

275g organic carrots	Half a beetroot (beets)
1–2 small organic eating apples	360ml filtered or mineral water

1 Simply put the ingredients in a NutriBullet or similar blender and blend!

Antioxidant Berry Burst Smoothie [child-friendly]

A handful of blueberries
A handful of strawberries
A handful of raspberries
A handful of spinach
A handful of kale
1 teaspoon chia seeds
1 teaspoon coconut oil
250ml cashew nut or other plant-based milk substitute of your choice

1 Simply put the ingredients in a NutriBullet or a similar blender and blend!

NOTE FOR PARENTS

This selection of ingredients will provide protein, carbohydrates, healthy omega-3 fats and fibre. Berries are considered to stabilize blood sugar levels, are nutrient-loaded, and bursting full of antioxidants.

- Blueberries contain vitamins K and C, fibre, manganese and iron, and are high in anthocyanins (antioxidants), which are nutrient dense.
- Strawberries contain vitamin C, folate, potassium, manganese, magnesium and dietary fibre; they are also high in antioxidants and polyphenols.
- Raspberries contain antioxidants such as vitamin C and quercetin (known to help with allergies), and have been shown to have anti-inflammatory properties.
- Spinach is high in niacin and zinc, as well as protein, fibre, vitamins A, C, E and K, thiamine, vitamin B6, folate, calcium, iron, magnesium and phosphorus. One of its many health benefits is that it helps maintain brain function, memory and mental clarity.
- Kale contains protein, fibre, vitamins A, C and K, the omega-3 alpha-linolenic acid, and folate, which is key for brain development.
- Chia seeds contain fibre, protein, fat, calcium, manganese and phosphorous along with zinc and vitamins B1, B2 and B3. They are the highest combined plant source of omega-3 fibre and protein; they help to support the body's natural detoxification pathways, repair cells, reduce inflammation and support a healthy digestive system.
- Cashew nuts are rich in vitamin B complex, which can help protect from anaemia and keep gums and teeth strong.

Drink Your Berries and Veggies! [child-friendly]

A handful of blueberries

A handful of strawberries

A handful of cherries, stoned

Raw vegetables: try small amounts of kale, spinach, carrot and/or beetroot (beets)

1 Simply put the ingredients in a NutriBullet or a similar blender and blend!

NOTE TO PARENTS

If you are able to conceal a small amount of parsley, garlic, ginger or turmeric within the juice, please do so! These are immune boosting and are easily masked by adding more of your child's favourite fruit or vegetables. They contain many bioactive compounds that have powerful medicinal properties, such as acting as a natural anti-inflammatory.

Tropical Fruit Vitamin C-Rich Smoothie [child-friendly]

A selection of fresh tropical fruit, e.g. mango, kiwifruit, pineapple

A handful of strawberries (or blueberries)

1 tablespoon oats (oatmeal)

6 walnuts (optional)

250ml almond, coconut or oat milk

---

1 Blend all the ingredients together until smooth and serve.

What to Drink (and What Not to Drink)

- Water is so important, not only because it transports nutrients to the brain, but also because it removes toxins and keeps you hydrated and able to focus and concentrate. Always send your child to school with a water bottle. Filtered, alkaline or mineral water is ideal. Daily recommendations vary but the following is a guide: 5 glasses (1l) for 5–8-year-olds; 7 glasses (1.5l) for 9–12-year-olds; 8–10 glasses (2l) for 13+ (and adults). You can also try infusing the water with slices of fresh lemon, lime, orange, cucumber or mint. Make a big jug (pitcher) and store it in the fridge.

- In terms of milk, I recommend goat's milk, or if you child is intolerant, try plant-based milk (such as oat, almond or A2 cow's milk, which is lactose free and easier to digest).

- Avoid sweet drinks. I recommend 100% fresh fruit drinks that are not made from concentrate, especially if your child doesn't eat fruit. Avoid fizzy drinks (soda), especially during the school week, due to their effects on blood sugar levels and their arguably addictive properties. There is some anecdotal evidence that apple juice may increase hyperactivity and there is clinical trial evidence that certain additives, flavourings and colourings in cordial or squash (juice concentrate) are linked to hyperactive and attention-deficit behaviours (see research published in *The Lancet* by McCann *et al.* 2007).

Lunch

Power Brain-Boosting Brunch at Home

SERVES 1–2

1 courgette (zucchini)

A large handful of kale

3–4 asparagus spears

1 red onion

A handful of cherry tomatoes

2 mackerel fillets (or sardines), smoked, tinned or fresh

Cayenne pepper

Chilli flakes

Olive oil

Juice of 1 lemon (optional)

2 sweet potatoes, peeled and cut into 2cm cubes

1 organic, free-range egg (optional)

1 Preheat the oven to 180°C/Gas Mark 4.

2 Wash and then season the vegetables and the fish with cayenne pepper and chilli flakes, olive oil and lemon juice.

3 Put the sweet potatoes in a Pyrex or ovenproof dish alongside the fish and bake for 10 minutes.

4 Add the other vegetables and bake for a further 5 minutes.

5 Add a free-range egg (simply crack this on top of the vegetables and bake in the oven), if extra hungry.

6 Serve and enjoy!

NOTE FOR CHEF

An alternative is to scramble 2 eggs as a side dish or pan fry alongside the vegetables. Serve on a bed of your favourite lettuce leaves. Smoked salmon (lox) or avocados are great alternatives to the mackerel or sardines.

Zesty Avocado Crush with Beetroot and Rosemary Crackers

FOR THE AVOCADO CRUSH:

2 avocados

2 limes

Chilli flakes (optional)

Cayenne pepper

Paprika (optional)

Extra virgin olive oil

FOR THE ROSEMARY CRACKERS (MAKES AROUND 24):

1 small beetroot (beets), peeled and grated

150g buckwheat flour

1 tablespoon dried rosemary, chopped

1 teaspoon salt

3 tablespoons coconut oil or butter, melted and cooled

2 organic, free-range eggs

1 For the avocado crush, scoop out the flesh of the avocados and crush with a fork, adding the lime juice, chilli flakes and a pinch of cayenne pepper and paprika. Drizzle with extra virgin olive oil and add more cayenne pepper as desired.

2 For the rosemary crackers, preheat the oven to 180°C/Gas Mark 4.

3 Squeeze a tablespoon of juice from the beetroot gratings into a bowl.

4 Add the flour, dried rosemary and salt into the bowl and mix together with the beetroot.

5 Add the coconut oil or butter to the eggs and whisk in a separate bowl.

6 Pour this into the dry mixture and knead into a dough. If necessary, add a little water.

7 Line a flat baking sheet with baking paper. Cut out another strip of baking paper the same size and place the dough between the two sheets and roll out into a 30cm square.

8 Cut the dough into 24 rectangular crackers with a sharp knife, and use the knife to wedge thin gaps between the crackers so they cook separately.

9 Bake for 15 minutes until golden and crispy. Flip halfway to make sure they cook evenly on both sides.

10 Serve with the avocado crush.

11 You could add some optional finger foods such as sliced peppers (bell peppers), cucumber and cherry tomatoes.

Spanish Omelette with Your Favourite Vegetables [child-friendly]

This delicious omelette only needs about 15–20 minutes preparation, with a total cooking time of around 35 minutes. It will stabilize blood sugar levels and provide a slow-release meal packed full of protein and nutrients that will keep you satisfied until your next meal. Add some salad or serve it alone. It will feed the whole family or it can be kept overnight for the next day.

SERVES 3–4

500g new or sweet potatoes (peeled), cut into 5mm slices

100g petit pois

2 red or orange peppers (bell peppers)

1 large red onion, finely chopped

2 large tomatoes, finely chopped

2 large garlic cloves, finely chopped

Olive oil

6 organic, free-range eggs

A handful of spinach leaves, finely chopped

Cayenne pepper

Paprika

Freshly chopped flat-leaf parsley for garnish

Brown or portobello mushrooms and/or chopped kale (optional)

1 Boil the potatoes and petit pois for 3 minutes, or until soft.

2 Fry the peppers, red onion, tomatoes and garlic in a little olive oil.

3 Whisk the eggs, add the finely chopped spinach and the spices.

4 Add the potatoes and peas to the frying pan with the peppers, onion, tomatoes and garlic for another 3–4 minutes. You could also add some sliced brown or portobello mushrooms and/or a handful of chopped kale.

5 Transfer the ingredients from the frying pan to the egg mix and stir. Add a pinch of cayenne pepper and paprika.

6 Heat up more olive oil in the frying pan, pour in the egg and vegetable mix and cook for a further 5 minutes.

7 Place the pan under a preheated grill for 5 minutes, until the omelette is firm and browning.

8 Leave to cool for a few minutes, transfer to a dish, sprinkle over the freshly chopped flat-leaf parsley and serve.

Spinach and Cheese Omelette [child-friendly]

SERVES 1–2

2 organic, free-range eggs

1 tablespoon olive oil

10g Provolone cheese or vegan alternative, cubed

Fresh spinach leaves, torn

1 Whisk the eggs in a bowl or beaker.

2 Heat the olive oil in a frying pan over a medium heat.

3 Pour in the eggs and leave for about 90 seconds to 2 minutes.

4 Flip the omelette over, place the cheese and spinach leaves on one half, and fold the omelette over.

5 Turn the folded omelette over for a further 30 seconds, then serve.

NOTE FOR PARENTS

- Spinach is a rich source of vitamins A and K, folate and potassium. It also contains vitamins C and B6. You can discreetly blend it into juices and sauces too!
- If you want to make this recipe entirely vegan, a Follow Your Heart Vegan Egg range is available in Tesco or Holland & Barrett (in the UK). Potential alternatives to chicken eggs include duck, goose or quail eggs.

Homemade Sweet Potato Hash Browns, Baked Mackerel and Roasted Vegetables [child-friendly]

SERVES 1–2

FOR THE SWEET POTATO HASH BROWNS:

150g sweet potato, peeled and grated

1 tablespoon olive oil or coconut oil

2 spring onions (scallions), chopped

2 garlic cloves, crushed

2 tablespoons gluten-free flour

1 tablespoon chia seeds

Salt and pepper

FOR THE BAKED MACKEREL AND ROASTED VEGETABLES:

Smoked or fresh mackerel fillets, broken up (allow 1 per person)

A handful of cherry tomatoes or tomatoes on the vine, halved or sliced

1 red onion, thinly sliced

1 sweet red pepper (bell pepper), thinly sliced

3–4 asparagus spears, a handful of chestnut mushrooms, half a courgette (as preferred)

A handful of cavolo nero

1 Place the grated sweet potato in a cloth and squeeze out any excess moisture.

2 Heat half the oil in a pan, and add the spring onions and garlic. Sauté for a few minutes then transfer to a bowl.

3 Add the grated sweet potato, flour and chia seeds, and season with salt and pepper. Mix together and form into 4 small patties.

4 Heat the rest of the oil in the pan and fry the patties for 3 minutes on one side. Flip over and fry for 2 minutes on the other side, until cooked through.

5 For the baked mackerel and roasted vegetables, preheat the oven to 190°C/Gas Mark 5. Place all the ingredients apart from the cavolo nero in a glass Pyrex or ovenproof dish with a little olive oil, season and bake for 10 minutes.

6 Stir in the finely chopped cavolo nero for the last 2–3 minutes.

NOTE FOR PARENTS

If your child is particularly fussy, fry or scramble a couple of eggs and serve with the hash browns. You could also blend some cooked mackerel into the hash browns.

Grilled, Sliced Free-Range Chicken with a Selection of Raw Vegetable Crudités and a Side of Hummus [child-friendly]

SERVES 1

Slow-roasted, free-range, pasture-raised organic (Breton) chicken or chicken breasts

Wholemeal or seeded pitta

1–2 carrots, sliced into batons

1 pepper (bell pepper), sliced

Half a cucumber, sliced

A handful of cherry tomatoes

FOR THE HUMMUS:

400g can chickpeas (garbanzo beans), drained

1–2 tablespoons tahini paste

Juice from a freshly squeezed lemon

1 garlic clove, crushed

80ml extra virgin olive oil or 3 tablespoons Greek yoghurt

Pinch of ground cumin

Himalayan pink salt (optional)

A little cold filtered or mineral water

1 Use a slow cooker to roast the chicken overnight until the meat is tender and falls off the bone. Carve the chicken into slices.

2 Warm the pitta in the oven for about 5 minutes and cut into slices.

3 Place the raw vegetables in a bowl or on a plate.

4 For the hummus, mix all the ingredients together in a blender, blitz, and season to taste.

5 Place the hummus in a bowl for dipping.

6 Let your child help themselves and enjoy!

NOTE FOR PARENTS

- Organic, free-range chicken is a good source of protein and is low in calories (around 102 per chicken breast). It also contains carbohydrates, vitamins and minerals.
- Hummus contains protein and is high in iron, folate, phosphorous and B vitamins.
- Carrots are an excellent source of beta-carotene, dietary fibre, antioxidants, potassium and vitamin K1. They are heart- and eye-healthy.
- Raw peppers (bell peppers) contain vitamin C as well as several phytochemicals and carotenoids such as beta-carotene, which have anti-inflammatory and antioxidant properties; they are also good for weight loss.
- Cucumbers contain minerals such as potassium, magnesium and silicon. They are also anti-inflammatory and contain vitamins K and B and copper. They are great for hydration and can help remove toxins from the body. They contain multiple B vitamins, including B1, B5 and B7 (biotin).
- Tomatoes are a great source of vitamin C, biotin, molybdenum and vitamin K. They are also a good source of copper, potassium, manganese, dietary fibre, vitamin A (in the form of beta-carotene), vitamin B6, folate, niacin, vitamin E and phosphorus.
- Wholemeal pitta bread is high in fibre and low in fat and contains iron, magnesium, phosphorus, selenium and calcium. (Check the amount of sodium if shop-bought.)

Turkey Lettuce Wraps [child-friendly]

SERVES 1

2–3 slices of roasted turkey or pan-fried fresh turkey meat

A handful of cherry tomatoes or tomatoes on the vine

1 red, orange or yellow pepper (bell pepper)

1 large iceberg lettuce leaf per person

Homemade or shop-bought organic hummus (see above for the homemade recipe)

1 For a warm dish, simply dice a portion of fresh turkey and fry alongside the tomatoes and peppers in a pan with a little olive oil.

2 For a cold dish, use slices of roasted cold turkey and sliced raw tomatoes and peppers.

3 Spread some hummus onto a large iceberg lettuce leaf.

4 Place the turkey and vegetables inside and roll into a wrap.

NOTE FOR PARENTS

These can also be used as part of a packed lunch for school.

- Ideally make sure the turkey is organic and free-range (pasture-raised) so you can avoid the *hidden* additives such as hormones, antibiotics or pesticides. Organic turkey tends to have less saturated fatty acids (and hasn't been fed on omega-6-rich soybean oil pellets) and a healthier protein ratio. Turkey contains the amino acid tryptophan, which is needed to produce adequate amounts of the neurotransmitter serotonin, which is critical for wellbeing and mood.
- You could also use Wild Alaskan salmon instead of turkey. Wild salmon is rich in brain-essential omega-3 fats that are known to help improve attention deficits and moods in children.
- Tomatoes are rich in lutein and lycopene; these can protect the eyes against light-induced damage.
- Please use orange and red peppers (bell peppers) as these are high in carotenoids and have high antioxidant properties.
- Hummus is a good source of protein and is high in iron, folate, phosphorous and B vitamins.
- Lettuce is a low GI food, which can help balance blood sugar levels.

Organic Bone Broth/Soup [child-friendly]

Bone broths are very nourishing and healing for the gut and are also very easy to make. They help to seal the gut and make a nourishing warm drink, or they can be used as a stock for soups or casseroles. The biggest benefit of bone broth is that it contains collagen, a protein containing amino acids that helps rebuild connective tissue and seals and heals the protective lining of the gastrointestinal tract.

SERVES 3–4

1 whole free-range, organic chicken or organic grass-fed beef joint (1.45kg)

2 carrots, sliced

2 celery sticks, sliced

2 tablespoons organic apple cider vinegar

1 Place the whole chicken or beef joint in a deep pot, and add the vegetables and organic apple cider vinegar.

2 Fill the pot with water up to about 5cm from the top, and cook on a low heat for about 24 hours. You can also cook this in a slow cooker overnight, until the meat falls off the bone.

3 The fat will rise to the top; it is up to you if you prefer to scoop it off, but there are health benefits in the fat, so do make sure to leave a little.

NOTE FOR PARENTS

- Bone broth is commonly recommended for treating leaky gut syndrome, a condition observed in children with Autism, ADHD and other learning differences. It is immune boosting and also used to help overcome food intolerances and allergies. It is also thought to be beneficial for joint pain. Bone broth is rich in glutamine, glycine, collagen and proline. The mineral content of bone broth helps the body to absorb calcium, magnesium and phosphorus.
- Carrots contain beta-carotene, dietary fibre, potassium, antioxidants, biotin and vitamins K and C. They have a wide range of health benefits including for cardiovascular, liver and eye health.

Lunch on the Move

Healthy eating can become a little problematic when you are on the road and travelling to different destinations. I understand this more than anyone, as at one stage of my life I could be in 20 countries a year! It's the perfect excuse to 'cheat' and waste money on over-priced sandwiches and processed junk food. My recommendation is simple: plan ahead!

Make a smoothie and a healthy delicious salad with your favourite ingredients. Here are some of mine: rocket (arugula) or baby salad leaves, spinach, finely chopped kale, tomatoes, red onion, orange pepper (bell pepper), hummus and beetroot (beets). Add some smoked mackerel and/or smoked salmon (lox). Add lemon juice, finely chopped garlic and balsamic or apple cider vinegar. Store in the fridge overnight and take it away with you – simple, healthy and delicious.

Main Meals

I am delighted to share this quote about the importance of fish for the brain by one of my favourite fish and seafood chefs, Rick Stein, who has also generously provided one of his classic recipes for you to enjoy:

> I really believe that fish is good for the brain – what our grandmothers taught us turned out to be true. In layman's terms, fish oil lubricates the brain and makes it far faster. We are what we eat. If you have a balanced diet you will be healthier and that must include fish. But despite this knowledge, we have found that although healthy options are always readily available, very few people choose to eat them. We should all be consuming more oily fish to improve our quality and length of life, especially where healthy brain function is concerned. A country's topography has a huge effect upon diet (and potential new market places). Japan is predominantly mountainous but surrounded by huge expanses of sea. You can't grow all the protein requirements of a modern nation like Japan on the side of a mountain, so that's why Japan eats so much fish.[1]

---

1 Reproduced from *World Fishing Magazine* (2013) by kind permission of Rick Stein.

Devilled Mackerel with Mint and Tomato Salad[1]

SERVES 4

4 x 350g fresh mackerel, cleaned and trimmed

40g butter

1 teaspoon caster sugar

1 teaspoon English mustard powder

1 teaspoon cayenne pepper

1 teaspoon ground coriander (cilantro)

2 tablespoons red wine vinegar

1 teaspoon freshly ground black pepper

1 teaspoon salt

FOR THE MINT AND TOMATO SALAD:

225g small vine-ripened tomatoes, sliced

1 small onion, halved and very thinly sliced

1 tablespoon fresh mint, chopped

1 tablespoon lemon juice

1 Preheat the grill to high. Slash the skin of the mackerel at 1cm intervals on both sides from the head all the way down to the tail, taking care not to cut too deeply into the flesh.

2 Melt the butter in a small roasting tin. Remove from the heat, stir in the sugar, mustard, spices, vinegar, pepper and salt and mix together well. Add the mackerel to the butter and turn over once or twice until well coated in the mixture, spreading some into the cavity of each fish as well. Transfer them to a lightly oiled baking sheet or the rack of a grill pan and grill for 4 minutes on each side, until cooked through.

3 Meanwhile, for the salad, layer the sliced tomatoes, onion and mint on four serving plates, sprinkling the layers with the lemon juice and some seasoning. Place the cooked mackerel alongside and serve, with some fried sliced potatoes if you wish.

2 This is one of Rick's favourite dishes, and is reproduced here by kind permission of BBC Books, *Rick Stein's Seafood*, first published in 2001.

Jerk-Spiced Seared Tuna with a Mango, Coconut and Pomegranate Salad[2]

SERVES 2

2 tablespoons Mama's Jerk marinade (or jerk marinade equivalent)[3]

2 x 225g tuna loin fillets

3 tablespoons coconut oil

¼ teaspoon salt

¼ teaspoon black pepper

2 teaspoons grated coconut

50g pomegranate seeds

80g diced mango

1 pack of freshly washed rocket (arugula) salad

1 Rub the marinade over the fish. Cover and chill for 20 minutes.

2 Heat one tablespoon of the coconut oil in a large non-stick pan over a medium-high heat.

3 Remove the tuna from the dish, discarding any excess marinade. Add the tuna to the hot pan and cook for 2 to 3 minutes on each side, or to the desired degree of 'doneness'. Remove the tuna, place on a cutting board, and slice into 0.5cm-thick pieces.

4 For the salad, combine the remaining coconut oil with the salt and pepper, grated coconut, pomegranate seeds and diced mango in a medium bowl, add the rocket and toss well. Divide the salad evenly between two serving plates and top with the tuna slices.

---

3 Kindly supplied by Adrian Luckie of Mama's Jerk.

4 See https://mamasjerk.com.

Chargrilled Jerk Chicken, Quinoa and Kidney Beans with a Sweetcorn and Red Pepper Salsa[4]

This dish consists of a juicy chicken breast spiced with Mama's Jerk dry rub seasoning and Jerk marinade, which is marinated for 24 hours prior to grilling. For a healthier way to serve the dish, this recipe uses quinoa with kidney beans instead of the traditional rice and peas.

SERVES 2

- 80g quinoa
- 40g kidney beans (from a tin)
- 2 x 170g free-range chicken breasts, butterflied
- 1 tablespoon coconut oil
- 1 tablespoon Mama's Jerk dry rub seasoning[5]
- 1 tablespoon Mama's Jerk marinade (or jerk marinade equivalent)
- ½ red onion
- 2 tomatoes
- 1 green chilli
- 1 lime
- 1 red pepper (bell pepper)
- A large handful of fresh coriander (cilantro)
- 120g sweetcorn

1 Boil a kettle. Put the quinoa in a saucepan with 400ml of boiling water, and simmer for 15 minutes, then add the kidney beans.

2 To butterfly the chicken, carefully slice through one side of each breast from the thickest part to the thinnest, being careful not to cut right through to the end. Open out the chicken breasts to resemble a butterfly. Place in a bowl with one tablespoon of oil, the jerk

5 Kindly supplied by Adrian Luckie of Mama's Jerk.

6 For those living in the US, alternative jerk seasoning such as Dunn's River or Walkerswood Traditional Jamaican Jerk Seasoning can be used.

seasoning, jerk marinade and a pinch of sea salt. Marinade in the fridge overnight.

3 Heat a griddle pan (or frying pan) to a medium-high heat, then add the butterflied chicken breasts and cook for 5–10 minutes on each side, or until the chicken is cooked through.

4 While the chicken is cooking, make the salsa: finely dice the half red onion and tomatoes, and finely chop the chilli. Mix together in a bowl with half of the juice from the lime, and season.

5 Dice the red pepper, roughly chop the coriander (cilantro) and drain the sweetcorn. Drain the cooked quinoa and kidney beans and stir through the red pepper, sweetcorn and half of the coriander. Season with sea salt and black pepper.

6 Spoon the red pepper and sweetcorn onto two warm plates, top with the chicken and serve the salsa alongside. Sprinkle the chicken with the remaining coriander (cilantro) leaves and drizzle over the remaining lime juice.

Hawaiian-Style Tuna Poke Bowl[6]

This delicious dish is a combination of four key elements: jasmine rice, a slightly spicy shoyu (soy sauce) dressing, a few fresh vegetables and raw, cubed tuna. The rest of the dish can be prepared while the rice cooks, making this an incredibly quick meal. You can use either yellowfin/ahi or albacore tuna. Albacore is much higher in omega-3 fatty acids and it's one of the best-known food sources of vitamin D.

SERVES 4

Jasmine rice (approximately 90g per person)

2 tablespoons black sesame seeds

½ to 1 large jalapeño chilli pepper

4 spring onions (scallions)

3 tablespoons natural shoyu (soy sauce)*

2 tablespoons rice vinegar

1 tablespoon fresh lemon juice

½ teaspoon freshly grated ginger

1 teaspoon sesame oil

4 small Persian cucumbers (or ⅓ of a large English cucumber)

2 small ripe avocados

2 fillets of wild Pacific yellowfin (ahi) or albacore tuna (140–170g each)

1 First, start your jasmine rice. In the 30 minutes it takes to cook and rest the rice, you can then prepare the rest of this recipe.

2 Gently toast the black sesame seeds in a dry skillet (or frying pan) over a medium-low heat until just fragrant, about 4 minutes. Set aside to cool.

3 For the dressing, mince the jalapeño chilli pepper, using some or all of the seeds, depending on how spicy you want the dish (I use half

7 Kindly supplied by Randy Hartnell of Vital Choice.

a large jalapeño chilli pepper with seeds, which is just a bit spicy but without too much heat).

4 Thinly slice the white and light green portions of the spring onions. Combine the jalapeño chilli pepper and spring onions in a large bowl and then add the soy sauce, rice vinegar, lemon juice, grated ginger and sesame oil. Whisk to combine.

5 Thinly slice the cucumbers and stir into the dressing and let rest. This gives the cucumbers a lightly pickled flavour.

6 Once the rice is cooked, divide it equally between bowls or plates. Cut the avocados into small pieces (about 1cm).

7 Cut the tuna into small pieces (about 1cm) and gently combine with the dressing. Spoon the tuna, cucumber and a bit of dressing over each bowl of rice, then top with avocado and garnish with the toasted black sesame seeds. Serve immediately.

NOTE

* To reduce the recipe's sodium content, simply use a low-sodium soy sauce.

Roasted Halibut with Fennel and Orange[7]

With a light, mild flavour and delightful texture, halibut is quite lean, yet rich in protein, omega-3s, vitamin D and magnesium. Halibut is the perfect 'blank canvas', fitting well with many flavours, and it roasts to moist, silky perfection. This recipe takes just 20 minutes from start to finish, and is big on flavour but low in calories.

SERVES 2

---

2 teaspoons organic extra virgin olive oil (plus enough to prep your baking dish)

1 fennel bulb (or 2 shallots or 1 onion)

1 clove garlic

1 orange

2 tablespoons Kalamata olives (or feel free to substitute with other olives or capers)

60ml white wine (or orange juice or lemon juice)

2 fillets of wild Alaskan halibut (110–170g each)

---

1 Preheat the oven to 200°C/Gas Mark 6.

2 Prepare a baking dish with a light coating of olive oil.*

3 Remove the stalks from the fennel bulb and reserve the tender fronds. Cut off the root end, remove the hard core from the centre, and thinly slice with a kitchen knife or mandolin slicer.

4 Heat the olive oil in a sauté pan over a medium heat. Mince the garlic clove and then sauté the fennel and garlic for 5 minutes, until the fennel softens and the garlic begins to brown. Season with salt and pepper.

---

8 Kindly supplied by Randy Hartnell of Vital Choice.

5 While the fennel is cooking, using a sharp paring knife, cut down the sides of the orange, removing all of the peel and white pith, leaving just the flesh. Then cut the orange into slices along the middle, into circular sections.

6 Halve the olives, making sure to remove any olive pits.

7 After 5 minutes, or when the fennel is tender, turn the heat up to medium-high, add the white wine and simmer for 1–2 minutes. Pour the fennel, wine and garlic mixture into the bottom of a baking dish.

8 Season the halibut with salt and pepper and place on top of the fennel mixture, then top with the orange segments and olive pieces.

9 Roast for 10 minutes or until the halibut is just beginning to flake. Enjoy!

NOTE

*** To keep clean-up to a minimum, feel free to use one pan. Sauté the fennel and garlic in an ovenproof pan, add the wine and let it reduce, then lay the seasoned halibut, orange slices and olives on top and roast in the oven.**

Thai-Style Broiled Salmon[8]

Combining prepared Thai chilli sauce with a few other pantry items transforms it into a lovely marinade for wild sockeye salmon. You can make your own chilli sauce, but you'll find several brands in the Asian section of most supermarkets. Starting with a prepared sauce makes the recipe a breeze, but always check the ingredients first! Serve your salmon with a simple cold peanut noodle salad (using rice vermicelli) or wholegrain rice (brown or red and black) and some braised bok choy, pak choi or sautéed greens.

SERVES 4

1 tablespoon natural tamari or soy sauce

Juice and zest of ½ lime

1 tablespoon freshly grated ginger

4 tablespoons Thai chilli sauce*

5–6 spring onions (scallions), thinly sliced

4 portions (110–170g each) of wild Alaskan sockeye salmon**

9 Kindly supplied by Randy Hartnell of Vital Choice.

1 Whisk together the tamari, lime zest and juice, grated ginger, chilli sauce and spring onions in a shallow baking dish with a lid. Nestle the salmon in the sauce skin side up, and leave to marinate for 30 minutes to 2 hours.

2 Preheat the grill to high and position a rack 20–25cm from the heating element. Line a baking sheet with aluminium foil.

3 Place the salmon on the baking sheet skin side down, top each portion with a bit of the remaining sauce, and broil until cooked to your liking (6–8 minutes). You can easily slide the skin off the salmon before serving.

NOTES

* Choose a chilli sauce with no added sugar or made with Stevia instead of sugar.

** Sockeye salmon has the firmest texture, but you could use any variety of wild salmon.

Silver Salmon with Spinach and Herb Pesto[10]

Wild Alaskan silver salmon is recommended because it is leaner than sockeye or king salmon. You can keep it moist by slowly roasting it at a lower temperature. If your salmon portions are skin-on, you'll find it easy to slip off the skin after roasting.

The beauty of the pesto recipe is that it's more of a kitchen-sink preparation – use 60g of any combination of fresh spinach and fresh herbs for a wonderful and nutrient-dense addition to the luscious slow-roasted salmon. This is an opportunity to use up leftover greens and herbs, such as spinach with fresh basil, Italian parsley and fresh tarragon – any combination will work well. A hint of tarragon and lemon zest add depth to the pesto. You can of course use pine nuts for the pesto if you prefer, but pecans make a wonderful change. Ideally use a food processor to make the pesto quickly and effortlessly. If not, you can also use a blender or a good, old-fashioned pestle and mortar.

SERVES 2

2 portions of wild Alaskan silver salmon (approximately 170g each)

80ml extra virgin olive oil plus 1 tablespoon

30g pecans

1 clove garlic

30g baby spinach

30g mixed fresh herbs (such as basil, Italian parsley, tarragon)

30g freshly grated Parmigiano Reggiano cheese

Zest of ½ lemon

Salt to taste

10 Kindly supplied by Randy Hartnell of Vital Choice.

1 Preheat the oven to 150°C/Gas Mark 2 and line a baking sheet with parchment paper.

2 Pat the salmon portions dry and place them on the parchment. Drizzle with a tablespoon of olive oil and season to taste with salt and pepper.

3 Roast the salmon for 15–18 minutes, until it reaches your desired level of 'doneness'.

4 While the salmon roasts, gently toast the pecans until they just begin to brown and become fragrant. You can do this in the oven or in a dry sauté pan over a medium heat (my preferred method). Remove from the heat and leave to cool.

5 Place the pecans, garlic, spinach, herbs, cheese, lemon zest and salt in the bowl of a food processor and pulse until finely chopped. With the processor running, drizzle in the olive oil and run until thoroughly combined. Season to taste.

6 Once the salmon is done, top each portion with a generous dollop of the pesto.

7 To store leftover pesto, press a piece of plastic wrap on the surface to prevent browning and refrigerate (use the following day).

Curried Cauliflower Soup[10]

Note from Tom Kerridge: 'I've eaten a lot of cauliflower on my low-carb diet and I've grown to love it. When it's cooked and puréed like this, it takes on such a rich, creamy texture that it feels quite indulgent, particularly when combined with the coconut and cream cheese. It takes on spices beautifully, too.'

SERVES 4

- 50g dried onion flakes
- 2 tablespoons vegetable oil
- 50g butter
- 1 onion
- 2 garlic cloves, grated
- 1½ tablespoons curry powder
- 1 chicken or vegetable stock cube
- 1 large cauliflower (about 800g), broken into florets
- 200ml coconut cream
- 200g cream cheese
- Sea salt and cayenne pepper
- 4 tablespoons chopped coriander (cilantro)
- 2 hot green chillies, sliced, seeds and all
- Finely grated zest of 1 lime

11 Reproduced with kind permission © Tom Kerridge (2017) *The Dopamine Diet*, Bloomsbury Publishing Plc.

1 Preheat the oven to 180°C/Gas Mark 4.

2 Scatter the onion flakes on a baking tray, trickle over the oil, give it a stir and season with salt. Bake for 5 minutes, or until the onion flakes are golden brown. Set aside to cool.

3 In a large saucepan, melt the butter over a medium-low heat. Add the onion and garlic and sweat gently, stirring from time to time, for 10–15 minutes, until soft.

4 Sprinkle over the curry powder and cook, stirring, for 2–3 minutes.

5 Now pour in 1 litre water and crumble in the stock cube. Bring to the boil and add the cauliflower florets. Turn the heat down to a simmer and cook for 5–10 minutes, until the cauliflower is soft.

6 Stir in the coconut cream and cream cheese until fully combined. Bring back to the boil then take the pan off the heat.

7 Blitz with a stick blender, or in a jug blender or food processor. If you've time, pass the soup through a sieve into a clean pan at this point – this will give the soup an unbelievably silky and delicious texture. Warm gently and season to taste with salt and cayenne pepper.

8 Ladle the soup into warmed bowls and scatter over the toasted onion flakes, coriander, chilli and lime zest.

Seafood and Courgette Soup

SERVES 3–4

2–3 large courgettes (zucchini) or leeks

2 medium-size tomatoes

4 garlic cloves

1–2 red chillies

440g white fish, from sustainable sources

Olive oil

1 sprig of thyme

400g prawns, mussels or clams (or other favourite seafood)

150g marinated artichokes

A bunch of sliced spring onions (scallions)

A spoonful of crème fraîche

1 Spiralize or chop the courgettes (or slice the leeks) and roughly chop the tomatoes. Finely slice the garlic and chillies. Chop the white fish into chunks.

2 Cook the courgettes or leeks, chilli and garlic in olive oil over a medium heat until soft.

3 Add 1 litre of water and bring to the boil, reduce heat and simmer until the vegetables are cooked.

4 Add the tomatoes and fish. Add the thyme when the fish turns opaque. Add the marinated artichokes, prawns, mussels or clams and cook until the prawns are cooked and the mussels open.

5 Season and serve with a drizzle of virgin olive oil or a spoonful of crème fraîche and finely chopped spring onions.

Steak, Red Onion and Tomato Salad[11]

Note from Tom Kerridge: 'I love beef and tomatoes together. The sweet acidity of the tomatoes combined with the salty, meaty crust on the steak works brilliantly in this salad. It's ideal if you want to get something really appetizing on the table quickly. Bavette, sometimes called skirt steak, has a fantastic flavour and is great value for money but it can be tough if you overcook it, so make sure you keep it nice and pink. Of course, you can swap the bavette for sirloin or rib eye if you prefer.'

SERVES 2

4 plum tomatoes, thinly sliced

1 small red onion, halved and thinly sliced

½ teaspoon cracked black pepper

Flaky sea salt

Vegetable oil, for cooking

2 bavette steaks (250g each)

20g butter

Juice of ½ lemon

1 ball of mozzarella (about 125g), drained and diced

½ bunch of basil (about 15g), large stems discarded

2 tablespoons sun-dried tomatoes, roughly chopped

1 red chilli, thinly sliced, seeds and all

1 tablespoon best-quality balsamic vinegar

¾ tablespoon extra virgin olive oil

25g Parmesan cheese, to finish

12 Reproduced with kind permission © Tom Kerridge (2017) *The Dopamine Diet*, Bloomsbury Publishing Plc.

1 Arrange the sliced tomatoes on a large serving plate. Scatter over the red onion, sprinkle with half of the cracked black pepper and season with salt to taste.

2 Heat a splash of oil in a frying pan over a medium-high heat. Season the steaks with salt and the remaining cracked pepper and place them in the hot pan. Add the butter and let it brown and colour the steaks well. This will take 4–5 minutes. Flip the steaks over and add the lemon juice and cook, basting the meat with the lemony butter, for 1–2 minutes.

3 Lift the steaks out of the frying pan onto a warm plate and leave to rest in a warm place for 10 minutes.

4 Drain off any liquid from the tomato plate. Scatter the mozzarella, basil leaves, sun-dried tomatoes and chilli over the tomatoes.

5 Slice the beef against the grain and arrange it over the tomato salad. Pour over any juices that have accumulated on the steak plate too.

6 Mix the balsamic vinegar and olive oil together and drizzle all over the salad.

7 Grate over the Parmesan just before serving.

Seafood Pesto Linguine

SERVES 4

Olive oil

2 Wild Alaskan salmon fillets

2–3 garlic cloves

Chilli flakes

Cayenne pepper

Juice from ½ a lemon

1 courgette (zucchini), finely chopped

1 red pepper (bell pepper), finely chopped

1–2 red onions, finely chopped

A bunch of asparagus, chopped

A handful of cherry tomatoes, halved

A handful of kale, chopped

225g spelt pasta of your choice or 4 large courgettes (zucchini), spiralized

Organic rocket (arugula) or mixed salad greens or baby spring greens

Balsamic or apple cider vinegar

Himalayan pink salt

FOR THE PESTO:

80g fresh basil leaves

120ml olive oil (add more if you need)

50g freshly grated Parmesan cheese

2 garlic cloves

50g pine nuts

Juice of 1 lime

1 For the pesto, blend all the ingredients for 2 minutes until a smooth paste consistency.

2 Preheat a pan with a little olive oil. Add the salmon, skin side up, and some finely chopped garlic, chilli flakes, cayenne pepper, a pinch of Himalayan pink salt and juice from half a freshly squeezed lemon. Cook for around 7 minutes.

3 Flip the fillets over and add the vegetables (courgette, sweet pepper, red onion, asparagus and tomatoes) and simmer for a further 7 minutes. Add some chopped kale for the last 2 minutes.

4 Prepare the pasta by placing it in a saucepan of simmering boiling water for around 6–8 minutes, then drain. Add the pasta and pesto to the vegetables, stirring for a minute or so.

5 Serve with mixed salad greens (rocket and spinach leaves are my favourites) and some balsamic or apple cider vinegar to taste.

NOTE FOR CHEF

Try also adding some pan-fried wild king prawns and scallops if you are a seafood lover like me. They only take minutes to cook with a little lemon juice, chopped garlic and olive oil. Add chilli flakes for a little extra spice.

Prawn Linguine [child-friendly]

SERVES 1–2

100g wheat and gluten-free linguine (or brown rice)

1 tablespoon butter or coconut oil

1 shallot, finely chopped

2 garlic cloves, crushed

100g cherry tomatoes, halved

2 tablespoons tomato puree

1 red chilli, finely chopped (optional)

250g prawns, raw

Olive oil

Salt and pepper

Rocket (arugula)

Balsamic vinegar or apple cider vinegar

Vegan parmesan flakes (optional)

1 Cook the pasta in slightly salted water.

2 Heat the butter or oil in a pan, add the shallot and sauté for 5 minutes, then add the garlic and a pinch of salt.

3 Stir for 30 seconds, then add the tomatoes, tomato puree and the chilli, stir well and cook for 2 minutes.

4 Add the prawns and cook until pink, then throw in the pasta, a splash of olive oil and a pinch of salt and pepper.

5 Serve with a side of rocket salad and balsamic vinegar or apple cider vinegar. You could add some vegan parmesan flakes.

Homemade Seafood Paella

This is one of my favourite comfort foods and super-nourishing, a dish both family and friends will enjoy!

SERVES 4–6

Free-range, organic chicken breasts (approximately 1 per person)

Red onions, tomatoes, asparagus, courgette (zucchini), orange and yellow peppers (bell peppers), finely chopped

3 cloves garlic

Saffron, chilli flakes, Himalayan pink salt, cayenne pepper

Olive oil

Short grain rice (approximately 90g per person)

Organic chicken and/or vegetable stock

Seafood (e.g. king prawns, scallops, muscles, clams)

A mixture of green leaves

1 If you eat chicken, I recommend choosing a free-range, Breton chicken. Place it in a slow cooker overnight so the meat literally falls off the bone, and then add it to the rice and vegetables when they are almost ready. The rice should be soft when cooked. (If you don't eat meat or fish, simply add more vegetables.)

2 Gently pan fry the chicken, vegetables, garlic and spices in the olive oil for a few minutes only, then add the rice and some of the stock, and keep adding the stock, allowing the ingredients to simmer gently for 25 minutes or so.

3 Make sure you add the scallops, prawns and other seafood during the last 4–5 minutes as they take less time.

4 Serve on a bed of succulent organic green leaves!

Sea Bass with Sweet Potato Wedges and Vegetables

SERVES 2

2 sweet potatoes

Olive oil or coconut oil

Paprika

2 sea bass fillets (approximately 90–100g per fillet)

1 garlic clove, finely chopped

Cayenne pepper (optional)

1 red onion, cut into wedges

Bunch of asparagus

A handful of cherry tomatoes

Spinach, kale or other green leaves

1 Preheat the oven to 200°C/Gas Mark 6. Peel, then cut the sweet potatoes into wedges, brush with olive or coconut oil and bake for 45 minutes to an hour. Sprinkle with a dusting of paprika.

2 Pan fry the sea bass fillets in a little preheated olive oil (skin side down) and finely chopped garlic (add a sprinkling of paprika and cayenne pepper or other seasoning of your choice if desired) for approximately 3–4 minutes. Then turn down the heat and add the onion, asparagus and tomatoes and cook for a further 4 minutes.

3 Serve on a bed of finely chopped spinach, kale or other succulent green leaves.

Pan-Fried Tuna on a Bed of Rocket with Roasted Tomatoes, Mozzarella Balls, Chopped Beetroot and Hummus

SERVES 2

1 tablespoon olive oil

Juice of 1 lemon

1 clove garlic, finely sliced (if you like spices, also use a small red chilli)

2 tuna steaks (approximately 240g per steak)

Balsamic vinegar or apple cider vinegar

Mozzarella balls

Rocket (arugula) or other salad greens (or extra fine green beans or asparagus)

A handful of cherry tomatoes, roasted

Chopped beetroot (beets)

Hummus (see the recipe for homemade hummus earlier)

1 Mix the olive oil and the juice of half a lemon with the garlic (and chilli if you want spice) in a pestle and mortar. If you like herbs you could also add coriander (cilantro) seeds or fresh basil. Smear over the fish.

2 Make sure the pan is hot first before adding the tuna steaks. Simply sear for around 1 minute each side, or cook for longer according to your preference. Season.

3 Add some balsamic vinegar or apple cider vinegar, the juice from half a freshly squeezed lemon and some mozzarella balls (sliced) to the rocket and serve with roasted tomatoes, chopped beetroot (beets) and hummus.

Baked Salmon Wrap with Sauté Potatoes [child-friendly]

SERVES 1

Wild Alaskan salmon (1 fillet per portion, approximately 85–115g each)

A handful of baby spinach leaves

Half an onion, sliced

Sprig of rosemary

1 lemon, sliced

Black pepper

175g new potatoes

Olive oil

Sea salt (optional)

A portion of vegetables to serve as a side (e.g. extra fine green beans, sweetcorn, carrots) or fresh salad leaves

1 Preheat the oven to 180°C/Gas Mark 4.

2 Place the salmon on a bed of spinach, add the onion slices, a sprig of rosemary and some lemon slices, wrap in baking paper and season with black pepper.

3 Bake the salmon for 10–12 minutes.

4 For the sauté potatoes: Place whole unpeeled potatoes in a pan of water. Bring to the boil and cook for 15 minutes. Drain and leave to cool. When almost ready to serve, strip the skins from the potatoes, and then cut into thick slices. Heat some olive oil in a large non-stick frying pan. Add the potatoes in a single layer if there is room, and cook for 10–15 minutes, turning them frequently with a fish slice until they are golden and crispy. Sprinkle with a little sea salt.

5 Serve the salmon and potatoes with extra fine green beans, sweetcorn, carrots or other vegetables of your child's preference or fresh salad leaves.

Homemade Fish (or Turkey) Burgers, Shoestring Sweet Potato Fries, Portobello Mushroom Buns and Carrot Slaw [child-friendly]

SERVES 3–4

4 boneless and skinless salmon fillets (550g total weight)

2 haddock fillets (or other fish, 250–350g per person)

Olive oil

4 medium-sized sweet potatoes

Ginger, freshly grated (optional)

Fresh lime juice

180g unrefined plain flour

2 organic, free-range eggs

2 slices of spelt bread (crumbed)

6–8 portobello mushrooms (2 per person)

Himalayan pink salt

1 tablespoon sesame seeds (optional)

FOR THE CARROT SLAW:

2 carrots, grated

Juice of half a lime

1 tablespoon olive oil

2 tablespoons natural dairy-free yoghurt

2 tablespoons sesame seeds

1 tablespoon fresh grated ginger (optional)

1 Preheat the oven to 200°C/Gas Mark 6.

2 Place the fish in a Pyrex or ovenproof dish with a little olive oil and bake for 8 minutes until cooked through.

3 Peel two of the sweet potatoes, cut into small pieces and boil. Alternatively bake the sweet potatoes in their skins at 200°C/Gas Mark 6 for 45 minutes, until soft inside.

4 Add the cooked fish to the sweet potatoes (if baked, scoop the potato out from its skin first) in a mixing bowl and stir together with a little cold water. Add the ginger and lime juice. Form the mixture into 4 large patties.

5 Place the flour, eggs and breadcrumbs into three separate bowls. Dip the patties in each bowl in turn, place on a greased baking tray and bake in the oven for approximately 20 minutes, turning over after 10 minutes.

6 For the shoestring sweet potato fries: Slice the remaining sweet potato into fine strips and place in a hot pan of pre-heated olive oil. Fry until crispy, turning over every 2 minutes or so.

7 For the portobello mushroom buns: Wash the mushrooms with cool water or wipe clean with a paper towel, remove the stems and drizzle with oil (add Himalayan pink salt, black or cayenne pepper and garlic for seasoning, or have plain as preferred). Sprinkle the sesame seeds on top of the mushrooms and roast at 190°C/Gas Mark 5 for 10 minutes.

8 To make the carrot slaw: Mix all the ingredients together.

9 Place the patty with the carrot slaw between the two mushrooms and serve with the shoestring fries on the side.

NOTE FOR PARENTS

- Salmon is a great source of the long-chain omega-3s that are essential for the structure and function of the brain. Omega-3s can also help improve attention deficits and mood in children.
- Haddock is low in calories and a great source of protein and essential vitamins and minerals, including the B vitamins, especially B12, which is needed for the formation of red blood cells and is essential for food metabolism.
- Sweet potatoes are loaded with phytonutrients, fibre, beta-carotene, vitamins C and B6, folate and potassium.
- Carrots are also an excellent source of beta-carotene, dietary fibre and potassium. They can help protect against night-blindness and may help lower blood cholesterol, and there is some evidence they might protect against cancer.
- Portobello mushrooms are macronutrients that contain very few calories and consist of protein, carbohydrates and fibre. They also contain selenium, which is known for its antioxidant properties; potassium, a mineral that can help lower blood pressure; phosphorus, which helps aid bone formation; and copper, which is an essential trace element that helps increase the absorption of iron, sodium and B vitamins.

Gluten-Free, Wheat-Free and Dairy-Free Cod Fish Fingers, with Homemade Chips or Mashed Potatoes and Vegetables [child-friendly]

SERVES 2–3

50g desiccated coconut

30g almond flour

½ teaspoon garlic powder

¼ teaspoon paprika

¼ teaspoon ground cumin

¼ teaspoon Himalayan rock salt

¼ teaspoon freshly ground black pepper

300g fresh cod

4 medium-sized sweet potatoes

Coconut or olive oil

1 Preheat the oven to 200°C/Gas Mark 6.

2 Mix the coconut and almond flour with the spices and seasonings.

3 Slice the cod into chunks and coat in coconut or olive oil before rolling the fish in the flour and spice mix.

4 Bake the fish for 10–15 minutes.

5 The chips (French fries) can easily be made using whole potatoes or sweet potatoes sliced thinly, tossed in olive oil and baked in the oven for approximately 30 minutes (you could also use some spices).

Spicy Chilli Served with Baked Sweet Potato

When I lived in Washington DC, I would host dinner parties for a group of dear friends who came from all corners of the world, and this particular recipe was always a treat, especially when the snow fell outside. It became known as my winter-warming spicy chilli. I would serve it alongside a baked sweet potato with a sprinkling of goat's cheese and a side of rocket, cucumber, spring onions and tomato.

SERVES 4

4 sweet potatoes (1 per person)

450g sirloin steak grass-fed lean mince

Olive oil

200–250g organic, chestnut brown mushrooms, sliced

2 large onions, chopped

2 orange peppers (bell peppers), finely sliced

1 small tin (approximately 200g) cooked red kidney beans

1 small red chilli, finely chopped

3–4 cloves garlic, finely chopped

Chilli powder, cayenne pepper and/or Tabasco (optional, for those who love spice)

Goat's cheese (optional)

A handful of rocket (arugula) and salad leaves, cherry tomatoes, diced cucumber, sliced spring onions (scallions)

Balsamic vinegar

Juice from half a lemon

1 Preheat the oven to 200°C/Gas Mark 6.

2 Bake the sweet potatoes in the oven for an hour or so, until soft inside with crispy skin.

3 Pan fry the mince with olive oil and some seasoning. Drain the fat from the meat once it has turned brown, then add to a big pot, stir in the vegetables and kidney beans. Add the chilli, garlic and any other seasoning, and simmer for 30 minutes.

4 Remove the sweet potatoes from the oven and cut in half. Serve the chilli in the middle of the baked sweet potatoes and sprinkle over the goat's cheese.

5 Serve with salad on the side: mix together rocket, salad leaves, cherry tomatoes, diced cucumber and sliced spring onion. Add a splash of olive oil and balsamic vinegar and the lemon juice.

NOTE FOR CHEF

For vegetarians simply omit the mince and increase the vegetables.

I recommend making a big pot of the chilli and freezing some for later.

Organic Beef Meatballs with Bolognese Sauce and Gluten-Free Pasta or Brown Rice [child-friendly]

SERVES 2

200g lean, organic, grass-fed beef steak (or turkey) mince

½ red onion, finely chopped

1 large carrot, grated (can either be added to the meatballs or blended and added to the sauce)

2 cloves garlic, crushed

Herbs/spices (optional) (e.g. black pepper, mixed Italian herbs, turmeric, ground cinnamon and/or ground cumin)

300g gluten- and wheat-free spaghetti (spelt pasta or brown rice are alternatives, if no intolerances are present)

Parmesan or goat's cheese (optional)

FOR THE BOLOGNESE SAUCE:

2 tablespoons tomato puree

400g organic tinned tomatoes

2 large handfuls of spinach, finely chopped (can be blended first to disguise, if needed)

230ml organic vegetable stock or bone broth stock

1 carrot, grated or blended

1 To make the Bolognese sauce, add the sauce ingredients to a saucepan and stir gently over a medium heat. Bring to the boil then reduce the heat and simmer for 10–15 minutes until the sauce has thickened.

2 Preheat the oven to 180°C/Gas Mark 4. Mix together the mince, onion, carrot, garlic and herbs and spices. Scoop out tablespoons of the mixture and roll into small meatballs or patties.

3 Place the meatballs in a glass Pyrex or ovenproof dish and bake in the oven for 20 minutes.

4 At the same time, boil a pan of water for the pasta or rice, cook until soft, then drain.

5 To serve, divide the spaghetti into bowls of equal portion sizes, pour the sauce over the spaghetti (or rice) and add the meatballs.

6 Sprinkle with Parmesan or goat's cheese.

NOTE FOR CHEF

Bolognese sauce is simple and easy to make so please avoid the often over-priced shop-bought varieties with their added sugar, sodium and preservatives.

Grass-Fed Beef Kebabs with Gnocchi [child-friendly]

SERVES 2–4

250g sirloin beef steak per person, cut into 2.5cm cubes (or another organic, free-range meat of your choice)

4 skewers

4–5 medium potatoes (Russet, Desiree or Yukon Golds)

2 tablespoons olive oil

½ teaspoon Himalayan pink salt

120g unrefined plain flour

1 Thread the beef onto the skewers and preheat a griddle pan to a medium-high heat. Cook for 5–7 minutes, rotating every minute until cooked.

2 For homemade potato gnocchi: Wash the potatoes but leave the skin on, and place in a large pan of boiling water. Cook for 20 minutes or so, but do not pierce once the skins are starting to flake away a bit; remove the potatoes and drain. Leave to cool slightly in a colander. Put them in a mixing bowl, and using a potato ricer or masher, mash them, adding the olive oil and salt and until they are smooth and lump free (the skin will remain inside the potato ricer). Add the flour to bring the dough together until the mixture is firm but slightly sticky. Roll the mixture on a floured surface to form a long log, just under 2.5cm in width. Slice into 2.5cm dumpling-style shapes.

3 To cook the gnocchi: Prepare a large pan of salted water, cover with a lid and bring to the boil. Once the water is boiling, add the gnocchi a few at a time. Very quickly, the gnocchi will float to the top, indicating they are cooked. Remove with a slotted spoon and place in a large dish with a little olive oil. Bring the water back to boil, add more gnocchi and repeat this step until all the gnocchi is cooked.

4 You can add a pesto or tomato sauce or simply some vegan cheese or butter to flavour.

5 Serve with vegetables or salad.

Chicken and Vegetable Risotto [child-friendly]

SERVES 2

1 tablespoon olive oil

1 clove garlic, crushed

200g Arborio rice (risotto rice)

Chicken breast, cut into small pieces

235ml organic chicken stock (choose a low sodium option)

Broccoli, chopped into florets

1 carrot, peeled and finely chopped

400g chopped tomatoes and/or 1 teaspoon tomato purée as required for taste

100g petit pois (fresh or frozen)

1 Pour the olive oil into a saucepan and add the crushed garlic. Stir together and add the rice, chicken and stock, broccoli florets, carrot, tomatoes and tomato puree.

2 Cook until the vegetables are tender and the chicken is cooked through, which will take approximately 20–30 minutes (add more stock as required).

3 Finally, add the petit pois and heat for 2 minutes, until gently simmering around the edges.

Roast Lamb with Oven-Baked Vegetables and Butternut Squash and Carrot Mash [child-friendly]

SERVES 4

1.5–2kg leg of lamb

1 garlic bulb

½ bunch fresh rosemary

1 lemon

Olive oil

Broccoli florets

Baby carrots

FOR THE BUTTERNUT SQUASH AND CARROT MASH:

110g carrots

½ medium butternut squash (about 600g)

Vegan milk

1–2 tablespoons vegan margarine (e.g. Pure) or olive oil (optional)

Salt and pepper

1 Preheat the oven to 200°C/Gas Mark 6.

2 Wash and then place the lamb joint in a large preheated ovenproof dish.

3 For the marinade, crush the garlic in a bowl, add the chopped rosemary, finely grate in the lemon zest, add the olive oil and then mix together, using a pestle and mortar.

4 Rub the marinade over the lamb, adding a little sea salt and black pepper if desired. Place the dish into the hot oven.

5 Cook the lamb for 1 hour 30 minutes for medium to well done, or less, as preferred.

6 For the butternut squash and carrot mash: Scrub or peel the carrots and chop them into small pieces. Cut the squash in half and scrape out the seeds using a knife. Take one half and peel off the skin with a potato peeler, then chop into small chunks. Place the carrot and squash in a saucepan and cover with water. Bring to the boil, then reduce the heat and simmer for around 20 minutes, or until both have become very soft when tested with a fork. Using a colander, drain the vegetables then return them to the saucepan. Use a potato masher and mash until smooth and creamy, adding a dash of non-diary milk to make slightly creamy. You could also add a little vegan spread or olive oil if desired. Mash until the mixture reaches the desired consistency. Add salt and pepper to taste.

7 Serve with broccoli florets and baby roasted carrots. The carrots can be added to the lamb for the last 30 minutes.

NOTE FOR PARENTS

- Lamb is a great source of protein; it also contains lots of vitamins and minerals including iron, zinc and vitamin B12.
- It is better to steam vegetables (especially broccoli) to retain as many nutrients as possible. Broccoli is rich in vitamins K, C, B6, E, B1, B2 and B3, omega-3 fats, zinc, iron and calcium, chromium (good for balancing blood sugar levels) and folate.
- Consider roasting parsnips, baby carrots and potatoes as alternatives to the mash if preferred.

Desserts

Tropical Fruit Salad[12]

SERVES 4

Half a pineapple

1 ripe mango

200g watermelon

1 papaya

2 kiwifruits

Lime juice from half a lime

1 small bunch fresh mint, leaves picked

1 tablespoon organic honey

200g low fat yoghurt

1 Trim the outside skin off the pineapple and cut out the hard core that runs down its centre.

2 Lay it on a chopping board and cut into chunks with a sharp knife. Place in a bowl.

3 Cut the flesh of the mango from the stone and scoop out the flesh from the skin with a spoon.

4 Cut the skin off the watermelon and dice into chunks, and place in the bowl with the pineapple.

5 Cut the papaya in half and scoop out the black seeds. Scoop the fruit out of the skin in the same way as with the mango, and place in the bowl.

6 Top and tail the kiwifruits, then, sitting each on one of its flat ends, trim the furry skin off with a sharp knife. Slice the kiwifruit and place in the bowl.

7 Drizzle the lime juice over the fruit.

---

13 Kindly supplied by Adrian Luckie of Mama's Jerk.

8 Take four plates and divide the fruit between them. Pound most of the mint leaves with the honey in a pestle and mortar. Spoon a little yoghurt over the top of the fruit on each plate and sprinkle over some of the mint sugar, add the rest of the mint leaves and serve.

Apple and Rhubarb Crumble [child-friendly]

SERVES 4

450g diced apple (or strawberries)

220g diced rhubarb

2 tablespoons orange juice

2 tablespoons honey

2 tablespoons flour (if gluten intolerant, use tapioca flour, e.g. tapioca starch)

½ teaspoon vanilla extract

FOR THE CRUMBLE TOPPING:

75g rolled or quick-cooking oats (oatmeal)

70g almond flour

3 tablespoons coconut oil (or butter)

3 tablespoons pure maple syrup (or honey)

1 teaspoon ground cinnamon

1 teaspoon vanilla extract

Salt

1 Preheat the oven to 180°F/Gas Mark 4.

2 Make the filling by combing the apple or strawberries, rhubarb, orange juice, honey, flour and vanilla, with a pinch of salt. Stir to combine and spoon into a baking dish.

3 Make the topping by combining the oats, almond flour, coconut oil, syrup, cinnamon, vanilla, and a pinch of salt. Mix with two forks or a pastry blender until well combined. If, after a few minutes, the mixture is still a bit dry, you can add a little more coconut oil or syrup. Crumble the topping over the fruit filling.

4 Bake for 40–45 minutes, or until the top is golden brown and the filling is bubbling. Leave to cool a little before serving.

Fruit Ice Cream [child-friendly]

SERVES 6

300g frozen banana

140g strawberries or blueberries

125ml dairy-free milk alternative (coconut or almond)

1 teaspoon maple syrup or Manuka honey

Nuts or seeds (optional)

1 This is a great alternative to processed ice cream. Simply blend the ingredients until smooth, place in a freezer-proof container and freeze overnight.

2 Serve in a bowl with a sprinkling of nuts or seeds (optional; make sure you always check for any allergies).

Chia and Strawberry Ice Lollies [child-friendly]

3 teaspoons chia seeds

250g ripe organic strawberries (blended)

100ml natural yogurt

1 teaspoon Manuka honey

1 Whisk all the ingredients in a blender and then pour into ice lolly moulds and place in the freezer.

Coffee, Chocolate and Chia Seed Pudding[13]

This is one of Tom Kerridge's guilty pleasures, which is only permitted when you have completed the first 28 days of my nutrition plan!

Tom's note: 'This is a very quick pudding – just mix it up and chill it in the fridge. The chia seeds make everything set to a soft, mousse-like texture. The pairing of orange and chocolate is always a winner and the coffee takes it to another level.'

SERVES 4

500g whole milk yoghurt*

70g chia seeds

1 tablespoon orange extract

2 tablespoons cocoa powder

20ml freshly made espresso

1 tablespoon erythritol (a sugar replacement)

About 2 teaspoons grated dark chocolate (80% cocoa solids)

About 2 teaspoons cacao nibs

About 2 teaspoons roughly crushed espresso beans

14 Reproduced with kind permission © Tom Kerridge (2017) *The Dopamine Diet*, Bloomsbury Publishing Plc.

1 Put the yoghurt into a bowl and whisk in the chia seeds, orange extract, cocoa powder, espresso and erythritol.

2 Spoon the mixture into four serving glasses, dividing it equally, and cover with cling film. Leave in the fridge for 12–24 hours.

3 When you're ready to serve, remove the puddings from the fridge and sprinkle evenly with the grated chocolate, cacao nibs and crushed espresso beans.

NOTE FROM DR GOW

* I also recommend coconut or almond non-diary milk.

Chocolate Chia Seed Pudding [child-friendly]

SERVES 4

- 250ml dairy milk alternative
- 40g chia seeds
- ½ teaspoon vanilla extract
- 1–2 teaspoons Manuka honey or maple syrup
- ⅛ teaspoon ground cinnamon (optional)
- Nuts or seeds (optional)

1 This pudding is a great alternative to processed ice cream. Simply blend the ingredients together until smooth and top with nuts or seeds and cool in the fridge for 1–2 hours before serving.

NOTE FOR PARENTS

- Chia seeds contain healthy omega-3 fats, vitamins A, B, E and D, and minerals, including sulphur, iron, iodine, magnesium, manganese, niacin and thiamine. They're also a rich source of antioxidants.
- The puddings can be pre-made and stored in the fridge for 2–3 days.

Healthy Snacks

- Prepare some raw vegetable crudités with a side of hummus. Experiment with carrot batons, sliced celery, sugar snap peas, radishes, cucumber, cherry tomatoes and red or orange pepper slices (bell peppers), and serve with rice cakes and hummus.

- Place some edamame beans with a little Himalayan pink salt in a bowl and serve.

- Prepare a selection of fresh fruit, e.g. grapes, blueberries, mango, sliced apples, orange segments, pear slices, pineapple chunks and cherries. These fruits are bursting full of vitamin C, an essential nutrient required daily as the body cannot store it. Vitamin C is key in the production of the neurotransmitter dopamine, which is vital for healthy brain development.

- Toasted wholemeal (gluten-free and wheat-free, if your child is intolerant) slices of sourdough or spelt bread with butter from grass-fed cows or dairy-free cheese spread or duck/chicken liver, mackerel or salmon pâté.

- A selection of nuts and/or seeds with optional pieces of dried fruit for older children. Mixed nuts contain zinc and increasing zinc consumption in children is linked to improvements in hyperactivity symptoms.

- Full-fat probiotic goat's yoghurt mixed with a small serving of grapes, dried mango, raisins or other fruit such as berries. Probiotic yoghurt contains healthy bacteria that can help to improve the balance of microflora in the gut, which are responsible for a healthy digestion. Healthy gut bacteria are linked to mood.

- Hot chocolate can be an occasional weekly treat; it is possible to make a sugar-free version by using 250ml of dairy-free milk alternative, 1 tablespoon of raw unsweetened cacao powder and 1 teaspoon of Manuka honey or maple syrup. Simply combine all the ingredients and gently heat in a saucepan.

Raw Cacao, Coconut and Hazelnut Balls

MAKES APPROXIMATELY 14–16

100g almonds or hazelnuts	100g coconut flakes
50g raw cacao	100g fresh dates
3 tablespoons coconut oil	Pinch of salt

1 Blend the nuts in a processor for around 1 minute or so.

2 Add the rest of the ingredients and blend for a further 3 to 4 minutes until completely mixed.

3 Roll the mixture into balls and place in the freezer for 20 minutes, then transfer to the fridge.

4 Serve with a glass of dairy-free, plant-based or goat's milk. Plant-based alternatives contain protein, calcium and iodine as well as vitamins C, D, B12, B2 and E. This can be warmed if the child prefers – stir while warming and heat for less than 5 minutes to avoid sediment building up.

Fruit and Nut Oaty Flapjacks

MAKES APPROXIMATELY 14–16

40g hazelnuts (always check for nut allergies)

300g oats (oatmeal)

50g raisins

50g cranberries

50g dried apricots

1 teaspoon ground cinnamon

1 teaspoon vanilla extract

120ml coconut oil, melted

1 tablespoon ground ginger

4 tablespoons organic honey

1 Preheat the oven to 175°C/Gas Mark 3.

2 Grease a baking tray with coconut oil and set aside.

3 Blend the nuts in a food processor, then add the rest of ingredients, including the coconut oil, and mix.

4 Pour the mixture onto the prepared baking sheet and bake for 25–30 minutes or until crispy on the outside and gooey on the inside.

5 Cool before cutting and serving.

NOTE FOR PARENTS

- Oats contain fibre and are rich in antioxidants. They are a slow-release food that helps stabilize blood sugar levels.
- Cranberries are immune supporting and contain antioxidants that can combat free radicals and pollutants. They also help protect cells from damage and are anti-inflammatory. They contain a range of vitamins and micronutrients including manganese, vitamins C, E and K, copper, fibre and pantothenic acid.
- Apricots are low in calories and an excellent source of vitamins A and C and beta-carotene. They also contain iron, zinc, potassium, calcium and manganese.

References

Abel, M.H., Caspersen, I.H., Meltzer, H.M., Haugen, M., *et al.* (2017) 'Suboptimal maternal iodine intake is associated with impaired child neurodevelopment at 3 years of age in the Norwegian Mother and Child Cohort Study.' *Journal of Nutrition 147*, 7, 1314–1324.

Adrian, R. (2008) 'From genes to brain to antisocial behavior.' *Current Directions in Psychological Science 17*, 5, 323–328.

Amen, D.G. (2013) *Healing ADD: The Breakthrough Program that Allows You to See and Heal the 7 Types of ADD* (Revised edn). London: Penguin Publishing Group.

Arnold, L.E. and DiSilvestro, R.A. (2005) 'Zinc in attention-deficit/hyperactivity disorder.' *Journal of Child and Adolescent Psychopharmacology 15*, 4, 619–627.

Baddeley, A. (1996) 'The fractionation of working memory.' *Proceedings of the National Academy of Sciences of the United States of America 93*, 24, 13468–13472.

Ballard, O. and Morrow, A.L. (2013) 'Human milk composition: Nutrients and bioactive factors.' *Pediatric Clinics of North America 60*, 49–74.

Barkley, R.A. (2014) *Attention-Deficit Hyperactivity Disorder: A Handbook for Diagnosis and Treatment* (4th edn). New York: Guilford Press.

Basset-Grundy, A. and Butler, N. (2004) *Prevalence and Adult Outcomes of ADHD. Evidence from a 30-Year Prospective Longitudinal Study*. London: Institute of Education, University of London: Bedford Group.

Bath, S.C. and Rayman, M.P. (2015) 'A review of the iodine status of UK pregnant women and its implications for the offspring.' *Environmental Geochemistry and Health 37*, 619–629.

Bath, S.C. and Rayman, M.P. (2016) 'Iodine: Food Fact Sheet.' British Dietetic Association (BDA). Available at www.bda.uk.com/resource/iodine.html (accessed 22 July 2020).

Bath, S.C., Steer, C.D., Golding, J., Emmett, P. and Ryman, M.P. (2013) 'Effect of inadequate iodine status in UK pregnant women on cognitive outcomes in their children: Results from the Avon Longitudinal Study of Parents and Children (ALSPAC).' *The Lancet 382*, 331–337.

Beard, J.L. and Connor, J.R. (2003) 'Iron status and neural functioning.' *Annual Review of Nutrition 23*, 41–58.

Beaumont, J.G., Kenealy, P. and Rogers, M. (1991) *The Blackwell Dictionary of Neuropsychology*. Oxford: Wiley.

Biederman, J. (1995) 'Psychoactive substance use disorders in adults with attention deficit hyperactivity disorder (ADHD): Effects of ADHD and psychiatric comorbidity.' *American Journal of Psychiatry 152*, 11, 1652–1658.

Bilicia, M., Yıldırıma, F., Kandi, S., Bekaroğlu, M., *et al.* (2004) 'Double-blind, placebo-controlled study of zinc sulfate in the treatment of attention deficit hyperactivity disorder.' *Progress in Neuro-Psychopharmacology and Biological Psychiatry 28*, 1, January, 181–190.

Birch, E.E., Hoffman, D.R., Castañeda, Y.S., Fawcett, S.L., *et al.* (2002) 'A randomized controlled trial of long-chain polyunsaturated fatty acid supplementation of formula in term infants after weaning at 6 wk of age.' *American Journal of Clinical Nutrition 75*, 3, 570–580.

Bjørkkjær, T., Brun, J.G., Valen, M., Arslan, G., *et al.* (2006) 'Short-term duodenal seal oil administration normalised n-6 to n3 fatty acid ration in rectal mucosa and ameliorated bodily pain in patients with inflammatory bowel disease.' *Lipids in Health and Disease 5*, 6.

Black, L.J., Allen, K.L., Jacoby, P., Trapp, G.S., *et al.* (2015) 'Low dietary intake of magnesium is associated with increased externalising behaviours in adolescents.' *Public Health Nutrition 18*, 10, 1824–1830.

Blasbalg, T.L., Hibbeln, J.R., Ramsden, C.E., Majchrzak, S.F. and Rawlings, R.R. (2011) 'Changes in consumption of omega-3 and omega-6 fatty acids in the United States during the 20th century.' *American Journal of Clinical Nutrition 93*, 5, 950–962.

Bloch, M.H. and Hannestad, J. (2012) 'Omega-3 fatty acids for the treatment of depression: Systematic review and meta-analysis.' *Molecular Psychiatry 17*, 12, 1272–1282.

Bloch, M.H. and Qawasmi. A. (2011) 'Omega-3 fatty acid supplementation for the treatment of children with attention-deficit/hyperactivity disorder symptomatology: systematic review and meta-analysis.' *Journal of the America Academy of Child & Adolescent Psychiatry* 50, 10, 991–1000.

Bondi, C.O., Taha, A.Y., Tock, J.L., Totah, N.K., *et al.* (2013) 'Adolescent behavior and dopamine availability are uniquely sensitive to dietary omega-3 fatty acid deficiency. *Biological Psychiatry 75*, 1, 38–46.

Bozhilova, N.S., Michelini, G., Kuntsi, J. and Asherson, P. (2018) 'Mind wandering perspective on attention-deficit/hyperactivity disorder.' *Neuroscience and Biobehavioral Reviews 92*, 464–476.

Breggin, P. (2007) *Talking Back To Ritalin: What Doctors Aren't Telling You about Stimulants and ADHD*. Lebanon, IN: Da Capo Press, Incorporated.

Bruce-Keller, A.J., Salbaum, J.M., Luo, M., Blanchard, E. 4th, *et al.* (2015) 'Obese-type gut microbiota induce neurobehavioral changes in the absence of obesity.' *Biological Psychiatry 77*, 7, 607–615.

Calder, P.C. (2010) 'The 2008 ESPEN Sir David Cuthbertson Lecture: Fatty acids and inflammation – From the membrane to the nucleus and from the laboratory bench to the clinic.' *Clinical Nutrition 29*, 1, 5–12.

Carey, N. (2012) *The Epigenetics Revolution*. London: Icon Books Ltd.

Casey, B.J., Jones, R.M. and Hare, T.A. (2008) 'The adolescent brain.' *Annals of the New York Academy of Sciences 1124*, 111–126.

Caspi, A., Williams, B., Kim-Chen, J., *et al.* (2007) 'Moderation of breastfeeding effects on the IQ by genetic variation in fatty acid metabolism.' *Proceedings of the National Academy of Sciences of the United States of America 104*, 47, 18860–18865.

Centers for Disease Control and Prevention (2020) 'National Diabetes Report 2020: Estimates of Diabetes and Its Burden in the United States.' Available at https://www.cdc.gov/diabetes/pdfs/data/statistics/national-diabetes-statistics-report.pdf (accessed on 2 September 2020).

Chalon, S. (2006) 'Omega-3 fatty acids and monoamine neurotransmission.' *Prostaglandins, Leukotrienes and Essential Fatty Acids 75*, 4–5, 259–269.

Chandler, S., Carcani-Rathwell, I., Charman, T., Pickles, A., *et al.* (2013) 'Parent-reported gastro-intestinal symptoms in children with autism spectrum disorders.' *Journal of Autism and Developmental Disorders 43*, 12, 2737–2747.

Cheuvront, S.N. and Kenefick, R.W. (2014) 'Dehydration: Physiology, assessment, and performance effects', *Comprehensive Physiology 4*, 1, 258–285.

Coe, C.L., Lubach, G.R., Bianco, L. and Beard, J.L. (2009) 'A history of iron deficiency anemia during infancy alters brain monoamine activity later in juvenile monkeys.' *Developmental Psychobiology 51*, 3, 301–309.

Colquhoun, I. and Bunday, S. (1981) 'A lack of essential fatty acids as a possible cause of hyperactivity in children.' *Medical Hypotheses 7*, 5, 673–679.

Conners, C.K., Goyette, C.H., Southwick, D.A., Lees, J.M. and Andrulonis, P.A. (1976) 'Food additives and hyperkinesis: A controlled double-blind experiment.' *Pediatrics 58*, 2, 154–166.

Conners, C.K., Levin, E.D., Sparrow, E., Hinton, S.C., *et al.* (1996) 'Nicotine and attention in adult attention deficit hyperactivity disorder (ADHD).' *Psychopharmacology Bulletin 32*, 1, 67–73.

Cordain, L., Eaton, S.B., Sebastian, A., Mann, N., *et al.* (2005) 'Origins and evolution of the Western diet: Health implications for the 21st century.' *American Journal of Clinical Nutrition 81*, 2, 341–354.

Cortese, S., Kelly, C., Chabernaud, C., Proal, E., *et al.* (2012) 'Toward systems neuroscience of ADHD: A meta-analysis of 55 fMRI studies.' *American Journal of Psychiatry 169*, 10, 1038–1055.

Costeira, M.J., Oliveira, P., Santos, N.C., Ares, S., *et al.* (2011) 'Psychomotor development of children from an iodine-deficient region.' *Journal of Pediatrics 159*, 3, 447–453.

Cryan, J.F. and O'Mahony, S.M. (2011) 'The microbiome-gut-brain axis: From bowel to behavior.' *Neurogastroenterology & Motility 23*, 3, 187–192.

Cubillo, A., Halari, R., Giampietro, V., Taylor, E. and Rubia, K. (2011a) 'Fronto-striatal underactivation during interference inhibition and attention allocation in grown up children with attention deficit/hyperactivity disorder and persistent symptoms.' *Psychiatry Research 193*, 1, 17–27.

Cubillo, A., Halari, R., Smith, A., Taylor, E. and Rubia, K. (2009) 'Fronto-cerebellar brain dysfunction in adults with childhood ADHD during sustained attention and reward.' *European Neuropsychopharmacology 19*, Suppl. 3, S303.

Cubillo, A., Halari, R., Smith, A., Taylor, E. and Rubia, K. (2011b) 'A review of fronto-striatal and fronto-cortical brain abnormalities in children and adults with Attention Deficit Hyperactivity Disorder (ADHD) and new evidence for dysfunction in adults with ADHD during motivation and attention.' *Cortex 48*, 2, 194–215.

Darwin, C. (1859) *On the Origin of Species by Means of Natural Selection, or Preservation of Favoured Races in the Struggle for Life*. London: John Murray.

Davis, N.O. and Kollins, S.H. (2012) 'Treatment for co-occurring attention deficit/hyperactivity disorder and autism spectrum disorder.' *Neurotherapeutics 9*, 3, 518–530.

Diabetes UK (2020) 'Facts and Figures.' Available at https://www.diabetes.org.uk/professionals/position-statements-reports/statistics (accessed on 2 September 2020).

Dillon, S. (2018) 'We learn nothing about nutrition, claim medical students.' BBC News, 25 March. Available at www.bbc.co.uk/news/health-43504125 (accessed 22 July 2020).

Dodig-Curković, K., Dovhanj, J., Curković, M., Dodig-Radić, J. and Degmecić, D. (2009) 'The role of zinc in the treatment of hyperactivity disorder in children.' *Acta Medica Croatica 63*, 4, 307–313.

Dougherty, D.D., Bonab, A.A., Spencer, T.J., Rauch, S.L., *et al.* (1999) 'Dopamine transporter density in patients with attention deficit hyperactivity disorder.' *Lancet 354*, 9196, 2132–2133.

Dunstan, J.A., Simmer, K., Dixon, G. and Prescott, S.L. (2008) 'Cognitive assessment of children at age 2½ years after maternal fish oil supplementation in pregnancy: A randomised controlled trial.' *Archives of Disease in Childhood – Fetal and Neonatal Edition 93*, 1, F45–F50.

Eaton, S.B. and Eaton, S.B., 3rd (2000) 'Paleolithic vs. modern diets – selected pathophysiological implications.' *European Journal of Nutrition 39*, 2, 67–70.

El Baza, F., Al Shahawi, H.A., Zahra, S. and Hakim, R.A.A. (2016) 'Magnesium supplementation in children with attention deficit hyperactivity disorder.' *Egyptian Journal of Medical Human Genetics 17*, 1, 63–70.

Evans, C.E.L., Hutchinson, J., Christian, M.S., Hancock, N. and Cade, J.E. (2018) 'Measures of low food variety and poor dietary quality in a cross-sectional study of London school children.' *European Journal of Clinical Nutrition 72*, 1497–1505.

Falony, G., Joossens, M., Vieira-Silva, S., Wang, J., *et al.* (2016) 'Population-level analysis of gut microbiome variation.' *Science 352*, 6285, 560–564.

Faraone, S.V., Perlis, R.H., Doyle, A.E., Smoller, J.W., *et al.* (2005) 'Molecular genetics of attention-deficit/hyperactivity disorder.' *Biological Psychiatry 57*, 11, 1313–1323.

Feingold, B.F. (1975) 'Hyperkinesis and learning disabilities linked to artificial food flavors and colors.' *American Journal of Nursing 75*, 5, 797–803.

Forsyth, J.S., Willatts, P., Agnostoni, C., Bissenden, J., *et al.* (2003) 'Long chain polyunsaturated fatty acid supplementation in infant formula and blood pressure in later childhood: Follow up of a randomised controlled trial.' *British Medical Journal 326*, 7396, 953.

Fox, K.C., Spreng, R.N., Ellamil, M., Andrews-Hanna, J.R. and Christoff, K. (2015) 'The wandering brain: Meta-analysis of functional neuroimaging studies of mind-wandering and related spontaneous thought processes.' *NeuroImage 111*, 611–621.

Freeman, M.P., Fava, M., Lake, J., Trivedi, M.H., Wisner, K.L. and Mischoulon, D. (2010) 'Complementary and alternative medicine in major depressive disorder: The American Psychiatric Association Task Force report.' *Journal of Clinical Psychiatry 71*, 6, 669–681.

Freeman, M.P., Hibbeln, J.R., Wisner, K.L., Davis, J.M., *et al.* (2006) 'Omega-3 fatty acids: Evidence basis for treatment and future research in psychiatry.' *Journal of Clinical Psychiatry 67*, 12, 1954–1967.

Funkhouser, L.J. and Bordenstein, S.R. (2013) 'Mom knows best: The universality of maternal microbial transmission.' *PLoS Biology 11*, 8, e1001631.

Georgieff, M.K. (2008) 'The role of iron in neurodevelopment: Fetal iron deficiency and the developing hippocampus.' *Biochemical Society Transactions 36*, Pt 6, 1267–1271.

Ghosh, S., DeCoffe, D., Brown, K., Rajendiran, E., *et al.* (2013) 'Fish oil attenuates omega-6 polyunsaturated fatty acid-induced dysbiosis and infectious colitis but impairs LPS dephosphorylation activity causing sepsis.' *PLoS One 8*, 2, e55468.

Gladwell, M. (2009) *Outliers: The Story of Success.* London: Penguin.

Golding, J., Steer, C., Emmett, P., Davis, J.M. and Hibbeln, J.R. (2009) 'High levels of depressive symptoms in pregnancy with low omega-3 fatty acid intake from fish.' *Epidemiology 20*, 4, 598–603.

Gow, R.V. and Hibbeln, J.R. (2014) 'Omega-3 fatty acid and nutrient deficits in adverse neurodevelopment and childhood behaviors.' *Child and Adolescent Psychiatric Clinics of North America 23*, 3, 555–590.

Gow, R.V., Sumich, A., Vallee-Tourangeau, F., Crawford, M.A., *et al.* (2013a) 'Omega-3 fatty acids are related to abnormal emotion processing in adolescent boys with attention deficit hyperactivity disorder.' *Prostaglandins, Leukotrienes and Essential Fatty Acids 88*, 6, 419–429.

Gow, R.V., Vallee-Tourangeau, F., Crawford, M.A., Taylor, E., *et al.* (2013b) 'Omega-3 fatty acids are inversely related to callous and unemotional traits in adolescent boys with attention deficit hyperactivity disorder.' *Prostaglandins, Leukotrienes and Essential Fatty Acids 88*, 6, 411–418.

Grantham-McGregor, S. (1995) 'A review of studies of the effect of severe malnutrition on mental development.' *Journal of Nutrition 125*, Suppl. 8, 2233S–2238S.

Grantham-McGregor, S. and Ani, C. (2001) 'A review of studies on the effect of iron deficiency on cognitive development in children.' *Journal of Nutrition 131*, 2S-2, 649S–666S; discussion 666S–668S.

Gurney, J.G., McPheeters, M.L. and Davis, M.M. (2006) 'Parental report of health conditions and health care use among children with and without autism: National Survey of Children's Health.' *Archives of Pediatrics and Adolescent Medicine 160*, 8, 825–830.

Haapala, E.A., Eloranta, A.-M., Venäläinen, T., Schwab, U., *et al.* (2015) 'Associations of diet quality with cognition in children – The Physical Activity and Nutrition in Children Study.' *British Journal of Nutrition 114*, 7, 1080–1087.

Hallahan, B., Ryan, T., Hibbeln, J.R., Murray, I.T., *et al.* (2016) 'Efficacy of omega-3 highly unsaturated fatty acids in the treatment of depression.' *British Journal of Psychiatry 209*, 3, 192–201.

Hawkey, E. and Nigg, J.T. (2014) 'Omega-3 fatty acid and ADHD: blood level analysis and meta-analytic extension of supplementation trials.' *Clinical Psychology Review 34*, 6, 496–505.

Helland, I.B., Smith, L., Saarem, K., Saugstad, O.D. and Drevon, C.A. (2003) 'Maternal supplementation with very-long-chain n-3 fatty acids during pregnancy and lactation augments children's IQ at 4 years of age.' *Pediatrics 111*, 1, e39–e44.

Hellström, A., Smith, L.E. and Dammann, O. (2013) 'Retinopathy of prematurity.' *The Lancet 382*, 9902, 1445–1457.

Hibbeln, J.R. (2002) 'Seafood consumption, the DHA content of mothers' milk and prevalence rates of postpartum depression: A cross-national, ecological analysis.' *Journal of Affective Disorders 69*, 1–3, 15–29.

Hibbeln, J.R. (2007) 'From homicide to happiness – a commentary on omega-3 fatty acids in human society. Cleave Award Lecture.' *Nutrition and Health 19*, 1–2, 9–19.

Hibbeln, J.R., Davis, J.M., Steer, C., *et al.* (2007) 'Maternal seafood consumption in pregnancy and neurodevelopmental outcomes in childhood (ALSPAC study): An observational cohort study.' *Lancet 369*, 578–585.

Hibbeln, J.R. and Gow, R.V. (2014) 'The potential for military diets to reduce depression, suicide, and impulsive aggression: A review of current evidence for omega-3 and omega-6 fatty acids.' *Military Medicine 179*, 11 Suppl., 117–128.

Hibbeln, J.R., Nieminen, L.R. and Lands, W.E. (2004) 'Increasing homicide rates and linoleic acid consumption among five Western countries, 1961–2000.' *Lipids 39*, 12, 1207–1213.

Hoogman, M., Bralten, J., Hibar, D.P., Mennes, M., *et al.* (2017) 'Subcortical brain volume differences in participants with attention deficit hyperactivity disorder in children and adults: A cross-sectional mega-analysis.' *Lancet Psychiatry 4*, 4, 310–319.

Huss, M., Völp, A. and Stauss-Grabo, M. (2010) 'Supplementation of polyunsaturated fatty acids, magnesium and zinc in children seeking medical advice for attention-deficit/hyperactivity problems – an observational cohort study.' *Lipids in Health and Disease 9*, 105.

Hynes, K.L., Otahal, P., Hay, I. and Burgess, J.R. (2013) 'Mild iodine deficiency during pregnancy is associated with reduced educational outcomes in the offspring: 9-year follow-up of the gestational iodine cohort.' *Journal of Clinical Endocrinology and Metabolism 98*, 1954–1962.

Iodine Global Network (2017) 'Global scorecard of iodine nutrition in 2017.' Available at www.ign.org/cm_data/IGN_Global_Scorecard_AllPop_and_PW_May2017.pdf (accessed 22 July 2020).

Isaacs, E.B., Fischl, B.R., Quinn, B.T., Chong, W.K., Gadian, D.G. and Lucas, A. (2010) 'Impact of breast milk on IQ, brain size and white matter development.' *Pediatric Research 67*, 357–362.

Jacka, F., Cherbuin, N. and Butterworth, P. (2015) 'Western diet is associated with a smaller hippocampus: A longitudinal investigation.' *BMC Medicine 13*, 215.

Judge, M.P., Harel, O. and Lammi-Keefe, C.J. (2007) 'Maternal consumption of a docosahexaenoic acid-containing functional food during pregnancy: Benefit for infant performance on problem-solving but not on recognition memory tasks at age 9 mo.' *American Journal of Clinical Nutrition 85*, 6, 1572–1577.

Kahan, S. and Manson, J.E. (2017) 'Nutrition counseling in clinical practice: How clinicians can do better.' *JAMA 318*, 1101–1102.

Kaliannan, K., Wang, B., Li, X.Y., Kim, K.J. and Kang, J.X. (2015) 'A host-microbiome interaction mediates the opposing effects of omega-6 and omega-3 fatty acids on metabolic endotoxemia.' *Scientific Reports 5*, 11276.

Kamal, M., Bener, A. and Ehlayel, M.S. (2014) 'Is high prevalence of vitamin D deficiency a correlate for attention deficit hyperactivity disorder?' *ADHD Attention Deficit and Hyperactivity Disorders 6*, 73–78.

Kerridge, T. (2017) *The Dopamine Diet*. London: Bloomsbury Publishing.

Knight, B.A., Shields, B.M., He, X., Pearce, E.N., *et al.* (2017) 'Iodine deficiency amongst pregnant women in South-West England.' *Clinical Endocrinology (Oxford) 86*, 451–455.

Knudsen, N., Christiansen, E., Brandt-Christensen, M., Nygaard, B. and Perrild, H. (2000) 'Age- and sex-adjusted iodine/creatinine ratio: A new standard in epidemiological surveys? Evaluation of three different estimates of iodine excretion based on casual urine samples and comparison to 24 h values.' *European Journal of Clinical Nutrition 54*, 361–363.

Kozielec, T. and Starobrat-Hermelin, B. (1997) 'Assessment of magnesium levels in children with attention deficit hyperactivity disorder (ADHD).' *Magnesium Research: Official Organ of the International Society for the Development of Research on Magnesium 102*, 143–148.

Kuipers, R.S., Luxwolda, M.F., Sango, W.S., Kwesigabo, G., *et al.* (2011) 'Maternal DHA equilibrium during pregnancy and lactation is reached at an erythrocyte DHA content of 8g/100g fatty acids.' *Journal of Nutrition 141*, 3, 418–427.

Landaas, E.T., Aarsland, T.I., Ulvik, A., Halmøy, A., Ueland, P.M. and Haavik, J. (2016) 'Vitamin levels in adults with ADHD.' *British Journal of Psychology Open 2*, 6, 377–384.

Lange, K.W., Reichl, S., Lange, K.M., Tucha, L. and Tucha, O. (2010) 'The history of attention deficit hyperactivity disorder.' *Attention Deficit Hyperactivity Disorder 2*, 4, 241–255.

Laufer, M.W., Denhoff, E. and Solomons, G. (1957) 'Hyperkinetic Impulse Disorder in Children's Behavior Problems.' *Psychosomatic Medicine*, January, 38–49.

Lee, T.H., Arm, J.P., Horton, C.E., Mencia-Huerta, J.M., *et al.* (1991) 'Effects of dietary oil fish lipids on allergic and inflammatory diseases.' *Allergy Proceedings 12*, 5, 299–303.

Levant, B., Radel, J.D. and Carlson, S.E. (2004) 'Decreased brain docosahexaenoic acid during development alters dopamine-related behaviors in adult rats that are differentially affected by dietary remediation.' *Behavioural Brain Research 152*, 1, 49–57.

Levin, E.D., Conners, C.K., Sparrow, E., Hinton, S.C., *et al.* (1996) 'Nicotine effects on adults with attention-deficit/hyperactivity disorder.' *Psychopharmacology (Berlin) 123*, 1, 55–63.

Liu, J. (2011) 'Early health risk factors for violence: Conceptualization, review of the evidence, and implications.' *Aggression and Violent Behavior 16*, 1, 63–73.

Liu, J., Raine, A., Venables, P.H. and Mednick, S.A. (2004) 'Malnutrition at age 3 years and externalizing behavior problems at ages 8, 11, and 17 years.' *American Journal of Psychiatry 161*, 11, 2005–2013.

Lozoff, B. (2007) 'Iron deficiency and child development.' *Food and Nutrition Bulletin 28*, 4 Suppl., S560–S571.

Lozoff, B., Beard, J., Connor, J., Barbara, F., Georgieff, M. and Schallert, T. (2006) 'Long-lasting neural and behavioral effects of iron deficiency in infancy.' *Nutrition Reviews 64*, 5 Pt 2, S34–S43; discussion S72–S91.

Lurie, A., Lurie, R. and Children's Hospital of Chicago (2019) 'Even the fetus has gut bacteria: Findings point to potential to improve preemie growth and immune system during high risk pregnancy.' *ScienceDaily*. Available at www.sciencedaily.com/releases/2019/10/191023132145.htm (accessed 7 September 2020).

Lustig, R.H. (2012) *Fat Chance: Beating the Odds Against Sugar, Processed Food, Obesity, and Disease*. London: Penguin Publishing Group.

Makrides, M. and Uauy, R. (2014) 'LCPUFAs as conditionally essential nutrients for very low birth weight and low birth weight infants: Metabolic, functional, and clinical outcomes – How much is enough?' *Clinics in Perinatology 41*, 2, 451–461.

Malito, A. (2017) 'Grocery stores carry 40,000 more items than they did in the 1990s.' Available at https://www.marketwatch.com/story/grocery-stores-carry-40000-more-items-than-they-did-in-the-1990s-2017-06-07 (accessed 7 September 2020).

McCann, D., Barrett, A., Cooper, A., Crumpler, D., *et al.* (2007) 'Food additives and hyperactive behaviour in 3-year-old and 8/9-year-old children in the community: A randomised, double-blinded, placebo-controlled trial.' *The Lancet 370*, 9598, 1560–1567.

McCann, J.C. and Ames, B.N. (2007) 'An overview of evidence for a causal relation between iron deficiency during development and deficits in cognitive or behavioral function.' *American Journal of Clinical Nutrition 85*, 4, 931–945.

McNamara, R.K. (2006) 'The emerging role of omega-3 fatty acids in psychiatry.' *Prostaglandins, Leukotrienes and Essential Fatty Acids 75*, 4–5, 223–225.

McNamara, R.K. and Carlson, S.E. (2006) 'Role of omega-3 fatty acids in brain development and function: Potential implications for the pathogenesis and prevention of psychopathology.' *Prostaglandins, Leukotrienes and Essential Fatty Acids 75*, 4–5, 329–349.

McQuaid, E.L., Kopel, S.J. and Nassau, J.H. (2001) 'Behavioral adjustment in children with asthma: A meta-analysis.' *Journal of Developmental and Behavioural Pediatrics 22*, 6, 430–439.

McVey Neufeld, K.A., Luczynski, P., Seira Oriach, C., Dinan, T.G. and Cryan, J.F. (2016) 'What's bugging your teen? The microbiota and adolescent mental health.' *Neuroscience & Biobehavioral Reviews 70*, 300–312.

Micallef, M.A. and Garg, M.L. (2009) 'Anti-inflammatory and cardioprotective effects of n-3 polyunsaturated fatty acids and plant sterols in hyperlipidemic individuals.' *Atherosclerosis 204*, 2, 466–482.

Moffitt, T. and Melchior, M. (2007) 'Why does the worldwide prevalence of childhood attention deficit hyperactivity disorder matter?' *American Journal of Psychiatry 146*, 6, 856–858.

Molteni, R., Barnard, R.J., Ying, Z., Roberts, C.K. and Gomez-Pinilla, F. (2002) 'A high-fat, refined sugar diet reduces hippocampal brain-derived neurotrophic factor, neuronal plasticity, and learning.' *Neuroscience 112*, 4, 803–814.

Montgomery, P., Burton, J.R., Sewell, R.P., Spreckelsen, T.F. and Richardson, A.J. (2014) 'Fatty acids and sleep in UK children: Subjective and pilot objective sleep results from the DOLAB study – a randomized controlled trial.' *Journal of Sleep Research 23*, 4, 364–388.

Monuteaux, M.C., Seidman, L.J., Faraone, S.V., Makris, N., *et al.* (2008) 'A preliminary study of dopamine D4 receptor genotype and structural brain alterations in adults with ADHD.' *American Journal of Medical Genetics Part B Neuropsychiatric Genetics 147B*, 8, 1436–1441.

Moshfegh, A., Goldman, J., Ahuja, J., Rhodes, D. and LaComb, R. (2009) *What We Eat in America, NHANES 2005–2006: Usual Nutrient Intakes from Food and Water Compared to 1997 Dietary Reference Intakes for Vitamin D, Calcium, Phosphorus, and Magnesium*. Washington, DC: US Department of Agriculture, Agricultural Research Service.

Mousain-Bosc, M., Roche, M., Rapin, J. and Ball, J.-P. (2004) 'Magnesium VitB6 intake reduces central nervous system hyperexcitability in children.' *Journal of the American College of Nutrition 23*, 5, 545S–548S.

Mousain-Bosc, M., Roche, M., Polge, A., Pradal-Prat, D., Rapin, J. and Bali, J.P. (2006) 'Improvement of neurobehavioral disorders in children supplemented with magnesium-vitamin B6. I. Attention deficit hyperactivity disorders.' *Magnesium Research: Official Organ of the International Society for the Development of Research on Magnesium 19*, 1, 46–52.

Mozaffarian, D., Lemaitre, R.N., King, I.B., Song, X., *et al.* (2013) 'Plasma phospholipid long-chain ω-3 fatty acids and total and cause-specific mortality in older adults: A cohort study.' *Annals of Internal Medicine 158*, 7, 515–525.

Neugebauer, R., Hoek, H. and Susser, E. (1999) 'Prenatal exposure to wartime famine and development of antisocial personality disorder in early adulthood.' *JAMA 282*, 5, 455–462.

Niederhofer, H. (2011) 'Association of Attention-Deficit/Hyperactivity Disorder and Celiac Disease: A brief report.' *Primary Care Companion for CNS Disorders 13*, 3.

NIH (National Institutes of Health) (no date) 'Sources of iodine.' Iodine Fact Sheet for Health Professionals, Office of Dietary Supplements. Available at https://ods.od.nih.gov/factsheets/Iodine-HealthProfessional/#h3 (accessed May 2018).

Nikolas, M.A. and Burt, S.A. (2010) 'Genetic and environmental influences on ADHD symptom dimensions of inattention and hyperactivity: A meta-analysis.' *Journal of Abnormal Psychology 119*, 1, 1–17.

Nogovitsina, O.R. and Levitina, E.V. (2007) 'Neurological aspects of the clinical features, pathophysiology, and corrections of impairments in attention deficit hyperactivity disorder.' *Neuroscience and Behavioral Physiology 37*, 3, 199–202.

Overtoom, C.C.E., Kenemans, J.L., Verbaten, M.N., Kemner, C., *et al.* (2002) 'Inhibition in children with attention-deficit/hyperactivity disorder: A psychophysiological study of the stop task.' *Biological Psychiatry 51*, 8, 668–676.

Partty, A., Kalliomaki, M., Wacklin, P., Salminen, S. and Isolauri, E. (2015) 'A possible link between early probiotic intervention and the risk of neuropsychiatric disorders later in childhood: A randomized trial.' *Pediatric Research 77*, 6, 823–828.

Peirano, P.D., Algarin, C.R., Chamorro, R., Reyes, S., *et al.* (2009) 'Sleep and neurofunctions throughout child development: Lasting effects of early iron deficiency.' *Journal of Pediatric Gastroenterology and Nutrition 48*, Suppl. 1, S8–15.

Perlmutter, D. and Loberg, K. (2013) *Grain Brain: The Surprising Truth about Wheat, Carbs, and Sugar – Your Brain's Silent Killers*. New York: Little, Brown & Company.

PHE (Public Health England) (2015) 'Composition of foods integrated dataset (CoFID).' 25 March. Available at www.gov.uk/government/publications/composition-of-foods-integrated-dataset-cofid (accessed May 2018).

Pulsifer, M.B., Gordon, J.M., Brandt, J., Vining, E.P. and Freeman, J.M. (2001) 'Effects of ketogenic diet on development and behavior: Preliminary report of a prospective study.' *Developmental Medicine & Child Neurology 43*, 5, 301–306.

Puri, B.K. and Martins, J.G. (2014) 'Which polyunsaturated fatty acids are active in children with attention-deficit hyperactivity disorder receiving PUFA supplementation? A fatty acid validated meta-regression analysis of randomized controlled trials.' *Prostaglandins, Leukotrienes and Essential Fatty Acids 90*, 5, 179–189.

Richardson, A.J. (2006) *They Are What You Feed Them: How Food Can Improve Your Child's Behaviour, Mood and Learning*. London: HarperThorsons.

Richardson, A.J., Burton, J.R., Sewell, R.P., Spreckelsen, T.F., *et al.* (2012) 'Docosahexaenoic acid for reading, cognition and behavior in children aged 7–9 years: A randomized, controlled trial (the DOLAB Study).' *PLoS One 7*, 9, e43909.

Richardson, A.J. and Montgomery, P. (2005) 'The Oxford-Durham study: A randomized, controlled trial of dietary supplementation with fatty acids in children with developmental coordination disorder.' *Pediatrics 115*, 5, 1360–1366.

Ríos-Hernández, A., Alda, J.A., Farran-Codina, A., Ferreira-García, E. and Izquierdo-Pulido, M. (2017) 'The Mediterranean diet and ADHD in children and adolescents.' *Pediatrics 139*, 2, e20162027.

Robinson, S.M., Crozier, S.R., Miles, E.A., Gale, C.R., *et al.* (2018) 'Preconception maternal iodine status is positively associated with IQ but not with measures of executive function in childhood.' *Journal of Nutrition*. doi:10.1093/jn/nxy054.

Rubia, K. (2007) 'Neuro-anatomic evidence for the maturational delay hypothesis of ADHD.' *Proceedings of the National Academy of Sciences of the United States of America 104*, 50, 19663–19664.

Rubia, K. (2011) '"Cool" inferior frontostriatal dysfunction in attention-deficit/hyperactivity disorder versus "hot" ventromedial orbitofrontal-limbic dysfunction in conduct disorder: A review.' *Biological Psychiatry 69*, 12, e69–87.

Rubia, K. (2018) 'Cognitive neuroscience of attention deficit hyperactivity disorder (ADHD) and its clinical translation.' *Frontiers in Human Neuroscience 12*, 100.

Rubia, K., Smith, A.B., Brammer, M.J., Toone, B. and Taylor, E. (2005) 'Abnormal brain activation during inhibition and error detection in medication-naive adolescents with ADHD.' *American Journal of Psychiatry 162*, 6, 1067–1075.

Sachdev, H., Gera, T. and Nestel, P. (2005) 'Effect of iron supplementation on mental and motor development in children: Systematic review of randomised controlled trials.' *Public Health Nutrition 8*, 2, 117–132.

Sagiv, S.K., Thurston, S.W., Bellinger, D.C., Amarasiriwardena, C. and Korrick, S.A. (2012) 'Prenatal exposure to mercury and fish consumption during pregnancy and attention-deficit/hyperactivity disorder-related behavior in children.' *Archives of Pediatrics and Adolescent Medicine 166*, 12, 1123–1131.

Salehi, B., Mohammadbeigi, A., Sheykholeslam, H., Moshiri, E. and Dorreh, F. (2016) 'Omega-3 and zinc supplementation as complementary therapies in children with attention-deficit/hyperactivity disorder.' *Journal of Research in Pharmacy Practice 5*, 1, 22–26.

Sanz, Y. (2010) 'Effects of a gluten-free diet on gut microbiota and immune function in healthy adult humans.' *Gut Microbes 1*, 3, 135–137.

Sarris, J., Kean, J., Schweitzer, I. and Lake, J. (2011) 'Complementary medicines (herbal and nutritional products) in the treatment of Attention Deficit Hyperactivity Disorder (ADHD): A systematic review of the evidence.' *Complementary Therapies in Medicine 19*, 4, 216–227.

Sarris, J., Logan, A.C., Akbaraly, T.N., Amminger, G.P., *et al.* (2015) 'Nutritional medicine as mainstream in psychiatry.' *Lancet Psychiatry 2*, 271–274.

Sayal, K., Prasad, V., Daley, D., Ford, T. and Coghill, D. (2018) 'ADHD in children and young people: prevalence, care pathways, and service provision.' *Lancet Psychiatry 5*, 2, 175–186.

Sears, B. (2008) *Toxic Fat: When Good Fat Turns Bad*. Nashville, TN: Thomas Nelson.

Shaw, P. (2013) 'ADHD: 10 years later.' *Cerebrum 11*.

Simopoulos, A.P. (2002) 'The importance of the ratio of omega-6/omega-3 essential fatty acids.' *Biomedicine & Pharmacotherapy 56*, 8, 365–379.

Simopoulos, A.P. (2016) 'An increase in the omega-6/omega-3 fatty acid ratio increases the risk for obesity.' *Nutrients 8*, 3, 128.

Sonuga-Barke, E.J., Brandeis, D., Cortese, S., Daley, D., *et al.* (2013) 'Nonpharmacological interventions for ADHD: Systematic review and meta-analyses of randomized controlled trials of dietary and psychological treatments.' *American Journal of Psychiatry 170*, 3, 275–289.

Spangler, R., Wittkowski, K.M., Goddard, N.L., Avena, N.M., *et al.* (2004) 'Opiate-like effects of sugar on gene expression in reward areas of the rat brain.' *Brain Research: Molecular Brain Research 124*, 2, 134–142.

Spedding, S. (2014) 'Vitamin D and depression: A systematic review and meta-analysis comparing studies with and without biological flaws.' *Nutrients 6*, 4, 1501–1518.

Sripada, C.S., Kessler, D. and Angstadt, M. (2014) 'Lag in maturation of the brain's intrinsic functional architecture in attention-deficit/hyperactivity disorder.' *Proceedings of the National Academy of Sciences 111*, 39, 14259–14264.

Stein, J. (2001) 'The magnocellular theory of developmental dyslexia.' *Dyslexia 7*, 1, 12–36.

Stein, R. (2001) *Rick Stein's Seafood*. London: BBC Books.

Stevens, A.J., Rucklidge, J. and Kennedy, M.A. (2017) 'Epigenetics, nutrition and mental health. Is there a relationship?' *Nutritional Neuroscience: An International Journal on Nutrition, Diet and Nervous System 21*, 9, 602–613.

Strazdiņa, V., Jemeļjanov, A. and Sterna, V. (2013) 'Nutrition value of wild animal meat.' *Proceedings of the Latvian Academy of Sciences. Section B. Natural, Exact, and Applied Sciences 67*, 4–5.

Stuss, D.T. and Alexander, M.P. (2000) 'Executive functions and the frontal lobes: A conceptual view.' *Psychological Research 63*, 3, 289–298.

Taylor, E., Dopfner, M., Sergeant, J., Asherson, P., *et al.* (2004) 'European clinical guidelines for hyperkinetic disorder – First upgrade.' *European Child & Adolescent Psychiatry 13*, Suppl. 1, I7–30.

Taylor, E., Sandberg, S., Thorley, G. and Giles, S. (1991) *The Epidemiology of Childhood Hyperactivity*. Oxford: Oxford University Press.

Trautmann, S., Rehm, J. and Wittchen, H.U. (2016) 'The economic costs of mental disorders: Do our societies react appropriately to the burden of mental disorders?' *EMBO Reports 17*, 9, 1245–1249.

von Stumm, S. and Plomin, R. (2015) 'Breastfeeding and IQ growth from toddlerhood through adolescence.' *PLoS One 10*, e0138676.

Watts, M. (2008) *Nutrition and Mental Health: A Handbook: An Essential Guide to the Relationship between Diet and Mental Health*. Brighton: Pavilion Publishing.

WHO (World Health Organization), UNICEF (United Nations Children's Fund) and ICCIDD (International Council for Control of Iodine Deficiency Disorders) (2007) *Assessment of Iodine Deficiency Disorders and Monitoring Their Elimination: A Guide for Programme Managers* (3rd edn). Geneva: WHO.

Wickens, A.P. (2004) *Foundations of Biopsychology*. Harlow: Pearson, Prentice Hall.

Wilens, T.E. (2004) 'Attention-deficit/hyperactivity disorder and the substance use disorders: The nature of the relationship, subtypes at risk, and treatment issues.' *Psychiatric Clinics of North America 27*, 2, 283–301.

Wilens, T.E., Faraone, S.V., Biederman, J. and Gunawardene, S. (2003) 'Does stimulant therapy of attention-deficit/hyperactivity disorder beget later substance abuse? A meta-analytic review of the literature.' *Pediatrics 111*, 1, 179–185.

Wilens, T.E., Vitulano, M., Upadhyaya, H., Adamson, J., *et al.* (2008) 'Cigarette smoking associated with attention deficit hyperactivity disorder.' *Journal of Pediatrics 153*, 3, 414–419.

Willatts, P., Forsyth, J.S., DiModugno, M.K., Varma, S. and Colvin, M. (1998) 'Effect of long-chain polyunsaturated fatty acids in infant formula on problem solving at 10 months of age.' *The Lancet 352*, 9129, 688–691.

Willcutt, E.G., Doyle, A.E., Nigg, J.T., Faraone, S.V. and Pennington, B.F. (2005) 'Validity of the executive function theory of attention-deficit/hyperactivity disorder: A meta-analytic review.' *Biological Psychiatry 57*, 11, 1336–1346.

Woolsey, T.A., Hanaway, J. and Gado, M.H. (2013) *The Brain Atlas: A Visual Guide to the Human Central Nervous System*. Oxford: Wiley.

Yap, J.J. and Miczek, K.A. (2009) 'Stress and rodent models of drug addiction: Role of VTA-accumbens-PFC-amygdala circuit.' *Drug Discovery Today: Disease Models 5*, 4, 259–270.

Yeh, T., Hung, N. and Lin, T. (2014) 'Analysis of iodine content in seaweed by GC-ECD and estimation of iodine intake.' *Journal of Food and Drug Analysis 22*, 189–196.

Yu, H.N., Zhu, J., Pan, W.S., Shen, S.R., *et al.* (2014) 'Effects of fish oil with a high content of n-3 polyunsaturated fatty acids on mouse gut microbiota.' *Archives of Medical Research 45*, 3, 195–202.

Zhou, F., Wu, F., Zou, S., Chen, Y., *et al.* (2016) 'Dietary, nutrient patterns and blood essential elements in Chinese children with ADHD.' *Nutrients 8*, 6, 352.

Zimmer, L., Delion-Vancassel, S., Durand, G., Guilloteau, D., *et al.* (2000) 'Modification of dopamine neurotransmission in the nucleus accumbens of rats deficient in n-3 polyunsaturated fatty acids.' *Journal of Lipid Research 41*, 1, 32–40.

Zimmermann, M.B. (2009) 'Iodine deficiency.' *Endocrine Reviews 30*, 376–408.

Acknowledgments

I am extremely grateful to my editor Amy Lancaster-Owen for her guidance throughout my first book writing and publishing experience. Thank you for embracing this important field of research and enabling the knowledge net to be cast far and wide. I hope we can publish many more books together. I would also like to thank Isabel Martin, Victoria Peters and all the team at Jessica Kingsley Publishers for their support and meticulous edits.

I am always filled with gratitude by the amazing guidance and mentorship I have received throughout the course of my academic journey. Professor Michael Crawford stands out as the single most influential guide in my life. His friendship and expertise have been invaluable. I must also thank Professors Eric Taylor and John Stein, and Dr Alex Richardson, whose help and support along my journey has both been humbling and heartfelt.

I am deeply grateful to copywriters Paul Sullivan (www.sullomeo.co.uk) and Keidi Keating (Book Angel) for proofreading, edits and revisions.

Above all, I thank all the families I have met during my career pathway and everyone who agreed to share their stories. A special thank you to Colman for stepping in and resolving my laptop issue at the last hour! I am also extremely grateful to the National Institutes of Health (NIH) for providing me with the opportunity to conduct cutting-edge research in an area I am so passionate about.

To all who have supported me in special, significant and varying ways: Bob Lister, the Mother and Child Foundation, Fran Peterson and Pamela Baker, Christopher Reid, Natalie Parker, Norris Windross, Kizzy Austin, Brandon Block, Charissa Saverio, Gary Francis, Patrick Jarrett, Rodney Lewis, Coco Das, Ana Cubillo, Hannah and Tim Sutton, the much-loved Troy-Bishop family (Mags, David, Charlie, Cydney Rose and Seth), all the Nutritious Minds Trust Ambassadors, Steve Tabakin, Emy P., Darrell Austin, Nigel Thompson, Lisa Nash, Paul Danan, Hayley Bassnett, Douglas Morrison and everyone who promotes the role of nutrition in brain health. A special thank you to Raymond Bingham for the large doses of serotonin, much laughter and his care and support.

Last but not least, I am grateful to my dear friend and mentor, Dr Brian Whittle, a remarkable scientist who was a huge advocate of the therapeutic effects of omega-3 fats (and cannabinoids). Brian knew I was writing this book but sadly passed away before getting to see it in print; this book is dedicated to his memory.

About the Author

Rachel V. Gow, PhD, is a child neuropsychologist, registered nutritionist (under the category of 'science') and neurodevelopmental specialist.

Dr Gow spent four years as a guest researcher in the Nutritional Neuroscience section at the National Institutes of Health (NIH) in Bethesda, Maryland. The NIH is considered the foremost biomedical research centre and an agency of the US Department of Health and Human Services. During her time at the NIH, Dr Gow co-designed and managed the world's first clinical trial testing the effects of omega-3 dietary fats in the brain function of adults with ADHD using neuroimaging techniques. The positive outcomes of this trial are expected to be published early 2021 and represent a novel contribution to the field of nutritional psychiatry. Dr Gow is also affiliated with leading academic and UK research institutions, namely King's College London and the University of Surrey in Guildford.

Dr Gow is a passionate advocate of brain health and has given lectures worldwide on nutritional neuroscience as well as interviews for television, radio and other media. She has also written many papers, articles and book chapters on the subject. Her PhD in Child Neuropsychology was awarded by the Department of Child and Adolescent Psychiatry at the Institute of Psychiatry, King's College London. Dr Gow had a first-class BSc in Psychology from Kingston University and an MSc from Birkbeck, University of London (graded Distinction). She has an active online presence and advocates for meaningful and positive change in children and individuals with ADHD and other neurodiverse conditions.

She currently lectures in psychology at London Metropolitan University and Nutritional Medicine at the University of Surrey. In her spare time she runs her non-profit (Nutritious Minds Trust) and sees clients at Nutritious Minds Consulting, a London-based (W1) clinic and partnership with award-winning doctor and psychiatrist, Dr Balu.

Dr Gow is the mother of an 18-year-old daughter and a 28-year-old son who received a childhood diagnosis of Dyslexia and ADHD at age nine. Her son was the driving force behind her career change from real estate to neuropsychology, and the original muse of this book.

Index